Living Well in a Nursing Home

Ordering

Trade bookstores in the U.S. and Canada please contact:

Publishers Group West
1700 Fourth Street, Berkeley CA 94710
Phone: (800) 788-3123   Fax: (510) 528-3444

Hunter House books are available at bulk discounts for textbook course adoptions; to qualifying community, health-care, and government organizations; and for special promotions and fund-raising. For details please contact:

Special Sales Department
Hunter House Inc., PO Box 2914, Alameda CA 94501-0914
Phone: (510) 865-5282   Fax: (510) 865-4295
E-mail: ordering@hunterhouse.com

Individuals can order our books from most bookstores, by calling (800) 266-5592, or from our website at www.hunterhouse.com

Project Credits

Cover Design	Peri Poloni, Knockout Books
Book Production	Hunter House
Developmental and Copy Editor	Kelley Blewster
Proofreader	John David Marion
Indexer	Nancy D. Peterson
Acquisitions Editor	Jeanne Brondino
Editor	Alexandra Mummery
Publicist	Jillian Steinberger
Customer Service Manager	Christina Sverdrup
Order Fulfillment	Washul Lakdhon
Administrator	Theresa Nelson
Computer Support	Peter Eichelberger
Publisher	Kiran S. Rana

Living Well in a Nursing Home

ss s

Everything You and Your Folks
Need to Know

LYNN DICKINSON, M.A., & XENIA VOSEN, PH.D.

with Severine Biedermann

Hunter House
PUBLISHERS

Hunter House Inc., Publishers
PO Box 2914
Alameda CA 94501-0914

Library of Congress Cataloging-in-Publication Data

Dickinson, Lynn, M.A.
Living well in a nursing home : everything you and your folks need to know / Lynn Dickinson and Xenia Vosen with Severine Biedermann.
p. cm.
Summary: "Concentrates on the positive aspects of nursing homes and offers strategies for identifying the best facilities—a guide for maintaining and improving relationships between the elderly and their families"—Provided by publisher.
Includes bibliographical references and index.
ISBN-13: 978-0-89793-460-2 (pbk.)
ISBN-10: 0-89793-460-1 (pbk.)
1. Nursing homes. 2. Nursing home care. 3. Long-term-care facilities. I. Vosen, Xenia. II. Biedermann, Severine. III. Title.
RA997.D496 2005
362.16—dc22   2005013624

Printed and Bound by Bang Printing, Brainerd, Minnesota
Manufactured in the United States of America

9 8 7 6 5 4 3 2 1   First Edition   06 07 08 09 10

Contents

🍎 🍎 🍎

Part II: You've Decided ... Now What?

Part III: Making the Most of Life in a Nursing Home

Important Note

The material in this book is intended to provide a review of information regarding nursing homes and other forms of long-term care. Every effort has been made to provide accurate and dependable information. The contents of this book have been compiled through professional research and in consultation with medical and mental-health professionals. However, health-care professionals have differing opinions, and advances in medical and scientific research are made very quickly, so some of the information may become outdated.

Therefore, the publisher, authors, and editors, as well as the professionals quoted in the book, cannot be held responsible for any error, omission, or dated material. The authors and publisher assume no responsibility for any outcome of applying the information in this book in a program of self-care or under the care of a licensed practitioner. If you have questions concerning the application of the information described in this book, consult a qualified health-care or mental-health professional.

Acknowledgments

❦ ❦ ❦

Every book is a collaborative effort. The authors would like to thank Spirit, God, or the Universe (whichever title you would prefer for the ultimate creative force) for bringing us together, bringing us to Hunter House, and assisting us in bringing this book to life with such extraordinary grace and ease and so much joy and laughter.

We'd further like to thank Jeanne Brondino, Kiran Rana, Alex Mummery, Kelley Blewster, and everyone else at Hunter House who had a part in making this project a reality and getting it into the hands of readers who need this information. Without the efforts of these people, this book might never have happened.

We owe our partnership with each other to Mark Victor Hansen and Robert Allen, whom we thank for providing the training we needed to make our ideas a reality. Without their enthusiastic mentoring, we would never have met. Special thanks go to Joycebelle Edelbrock and Denise Michaels. Without their advice and encouragement, this project would still be just another idea scrawled on a luncheon napkin.

Thanks to Lisa Nalewak and David Etheredge at Savvy Dog Communications. Without their keen design and marketing sensibilities, Hunter House might never have noticed this special little project.

We owe much to Severine Biedermann. Her long hours of research support, many conceptual contributions, and hands-on work made the entire project more feasible and bearable. Thank you, Severine.

Lynn would like to thank Clyde Smith and Aspen Smith for their loving patience and support while the book was being written, and David and Tracy Story and Elaine Hazlett for all the extra favors and assistance during the writing process. She'd also like to thank Drs. Ron and Mary Hulnick for their loving support, their sage advice, and the impressive level of life-mastery skills they so consistently demonstrate.

Xenia extends her appreciation to her whole nursing home team, and especially to Wolfgang Wagner, Heike Gerstel, Daniela Schwarzer, Irene Schneider, and Christina John, who did excellent work while Xenia was busy with the manuscript. Their enthusiastic interest in this book was both supportive and encouraging. Special thanks to Dr. Harald Thomas for his participation and encouragement, and to Dr. Marcel Boetschi for his spiritual support. Thanks also to Heide Schröder, Anne Wiedemann, and all the others who kept everyday life going during Xenia's visits to the United States. And, of course, special thanks to Jan Neersoe, who for more than twenty years has accompanied Xenia on her publishing journey with vital interest.

But most of all we owe our thanks to all the wonderful old people who taught us that living well in a nursing home is indeed a realistic possibility—every day and everywhere.

Preface

❧ ❧ ❧

... FROM LYNN DICKINSON

Why would anyone in her right mind want to write a positive book about nursing homes? Are there even enough good things to say to fill an entire book?

When Xenia and I first met, at a conference in Orlando, Florida, I was a business success coach who had never set foot in a nursing home, and she was a social gerontologist who had worked in the long-term-care field for more than thirty years. I was drawn to her bright smile and upbeat, friendly manner right away. I was surprised to learn that, of all things, she was the owner of several nursing homes. I could feel myself shudder as she told me what she did for a living. I remember wrinkling my nose at the idea of spending any time at all, even time at work, in a nursing home. I thought, *Oh well, she seems like a nice person anyway,* and figured we'd soon change the subject.

But over the course of our lunches during that week in January 2004, Xenia began sharing stories of nursing home life she'd collected during more than thirty years of working with elderly people. I was surprised at how many of her stories were interesting, uplifting, or amusing. She told of the nursing home staff trying hard to come up with just the right words to communicate with a patient suffering from dementia. Often a senile patient will no longer recognize words he or she learned as an adult, but will respond readily to words learned as a child. So, for example, asking a patient if he or she needs to "use the restroom" may be confusing, while asking if he or she needs to "go potty" or "go pee-pee" may yield a better result. She told of dedicated staff members trying word after word with their patients, until they found just the right one. I was struck by how positive Xenia's stories were. They illustrated a quality of care I had never imagined, having been subjected to our culture's common assumptions that nursing homes are associated with negativity, guilt, warnings, and lawsuits.

Knowing that every year millions of families struggle with the nursing home decision, and believing that there are at least two sides to every issue, I suggested that Xenia and I write a book together about the positive aspects of nursing homes—one designed to help people see the other side of the coin. I also wanted to help people see that their preconceptions may be the only things standing between them and a positive experience. The nursing home decision, like so many other events in life, is neither good nor bad, but, to quote Shakespeare, "thinking makes it so." It's time to stop reflexively being "against" nursing homes, as our culture seems to be. It's time to stop suffering unnecessarily when faced with the decision about what to do for a loved one's long-term care.

Of course, now that the book is written, I know a lot more about nursing homes than I did during that January in Orlando, and I feel a lot better about them, too. Choosing a nursing home is a tough decision to make, and there is plenty of negative information out there that can cause you to feel bad about your choices. We want to show you the other side of the nursing home picture— the side that will reassure you and will give you confidence that what you are doing really is the best you can do.

Santa Monica, California
July 2005

... FROM XENIA VOSEN

I am a social gerontologist. For over thirty years, I have worked in the field and have taught about the psychological and sociological aspects of aging, the problems and issues people face. However, working as a scientist and teacher was not enough for me. In 1992 I founded the first of my own nursing homes, reducing the gap between theory and practice and putting myself once again into the role of student. The opportunity to filter everything I had been teaching through the lens of the everyday practitioner was very beneficial. I often felt that the practical experience was more valuable than anything I had learned at university.

While I was playing the roles of teacher, scientist, and nursing home director, my role of daughter to a mother in her late eighties who had senile dementia grew increasingly important. During the last seven years before her death, my mother lived in one of my nursing homes, and so I found myself in yet another role: that of family member of a nursing home resident.

Last but not least, I myself grew older. I was no longer reporting on other people's problems, but instead had started asking, "What does all this have to do with me? With my future? With my emotions, hopes, and fears?"

Then I met Lynn Dickinson. Her reaction when she learned of my profession was the typical one: "Oh, that must be such an awful job!" An awful job? Oh no. Not at all. "Working in a nursing home is the most fulfilling job I can imagine," I told her.

This piqued Lynn's curiosity and triggered questions. I told her all about the fears of the old people and their family members, and I explained why those fears can be so damaging and so senseless. I told her story after story to illustrate what can make nursing home life a special, positive experience. "This news could be very helpful for a lot of people with older parents. Let's write a book and share those positive experiences!" Lynn suggested. I agreed, but only hesitantly, because I was busy with other projects at the time. Heaven must have sensed my hesitation and sent Severine Biedermann, a young author just starting her career, who had both the time for writing and doing research and the necessary sensitivity about the subject. Her open-minded questions, her curiosity, and her empathy for older people proved extremely helpful and encouraging.

While working on this book, I grew more and more convinced that it could be—no, that it *will* be—a great help for the many family members who phone us at the nursing homes in fear and despair, all with the same dilemma: "I urgently need a place for my loved one." It will be an anchor for those who enter such conversations feeling negative, even adversarial. May we end these conversations as partners, or even friends, working toward the same goal: a loving solution. Let us work together to make the last period in the lives of our loved ones as fulfilling and agreeable, as warm and caring, as humanly possible!

Bopfingen, Germany
July 2005

Introduction

❧ ❧ ❧

You are holding in your hands the first book to take a thorough look at the *positive* aspects of nursing homes. Yes, there are many. Even though you may not hear about them on the evening news, the positive aspects of nursing homes far outnumber the negative ones. And that is good news! As we write this, there are more than 1.6 million nursing home residents in the United States and nearly 3 million in the Western world. It is projected that within the next thirty years, there will be 5 million nursing home residents in the United States alone!

Why We Wrote This Book

First, it is important to clarify that the term "nursing home" is being used here as an umbrella term to cover a wide range of long-term-care options and facilities. We explain the different types of nursing homes more clearly starting on page 120.

Most of us think of nursing homes as a necessary evil to be avoided if at all possible. Increasingly, this belief does not serve us well. Although life in a nursing home is rarely considered a first choice, there are times when it may be a very good choice. For people who have been living independently for decades but who no longer have the mobility to do their own shopping, or who have become restricted in their social contacts, or who need assistance with basic activities such as dressing or meal preparation, life in a long-term-care facility, such as a nursing home or assisted-living program, may very well be the *best* choice. Still, arriving at the decision to place a loved one in a nursing home (or to enter a nursing home oneself) is usually not an easy one. The resident-to-be may feel angry, betrayed, victimized, or unloved. The decision maker

1

may feel guilty, anxious, obligated, or resentful. Part of the reason why we wrote this book is because we believe all this suffering is unnecessary.

This book takes a look at when it may be useful to start thinking about a long-term-care solution for yourself or a family member. If you are considering the possibility of caring for your loved one at home, we walk you through the process of making that decision so you will be aware of all the factors involved. We tell you what life in a nursing home can be like and give you some guidelines for choosing the appropriate type of facility for yourself or a loved one. We outline ways to discover and avoid the hidden problems in some nursing homes. We offer suggestions for working with nursing home staff to help ensure that you or your loved one is well cared for. We help you identify and cope with the inner demons such as guilt, anxiety, and anger that can act as barriers to peaceful and satisfying relationships between family members, residents, and nursing home staff.

We also wrote this book to assist you *after* you or your loved one has become a nursing home resident. Once the nursing home decision has been made, everyday life in the institution must be managed and optimized. A wide variety of issues and potentials for conflict arise. We discuss ways to deal with these so that your experience can be as satisfying as possible.

Who This Book Is For

Don't let the book's subtitle—*Everything You and Your Folks Need to Know*—fool you. This book is not just about elderly parents. Although we use the words "mother," "father," and "parents" in the examples throughout the text, you can apply what you learn here to a spouse, a stepparent, a grandparent, a neighbor, a friend, or any other loved one who may need your care and assistance in his or her later years. If you are considering moving into a nursing home yourself, you will find the information in this book extremely valuable. This book is for you and anyone else you know who is involved in any way with the nursing home decision and its aftereffects. It is for parents, spouses, siblings, older children, and even friends and neighbors who you think may have something to say about the decision—for better or for worse. Give a copy to everyone concerned, and the situation will be easier to handle all the way around.

Specifically, this book is for you if—

* your elderly parent or another loved one needs help with the normal activities of daily living, and you are not quite sure what to do

* you have decided to move your elderly parent or loved one into a nursing home or other long-term-care facility, but you don't feel very good about the decision—you are not absolutely certain you are doing the right thing

* you are in the process of searching for a quality long-term-care facility for your loved one, and you want to be sure you're choosing the right type of facility for his or her needs and your situation

* you want to know how to compare the various long-term-care facilities you're considering in order to choose the best home for your loved one

* your loved one already lives in a nursing home, and you are hoping to make the experience a better one for you, for him or her, and for everyone else concerned

* your elderly parent needs care, and you are considering bringing him or her into your home to live with you

* you are considering making the move into a long-term-care facility yourself

* you have a friend going through this transition with his or her own parents and you want to be supportive, understanding, and informed

And, finally, this book is for you if—

* you are an employee or administrator of a nursing home or other long-term-care facility, or are considering becoming one

Throughout the book we will introduce you to a number of real people who have made the elder-care decision on behalf of themselves or a loved one. We will also take you into everyday life in various long-term-care situations and introduce you to some wonderful older people. You can learn from their stories and decide for yourself what is best for you.

How to Read This Book

The book is structured in three parts to help you at various stages in your journey.

Part I, "Making the Long-Term-Care Decision," will assist you in clarifying your situation and show you some ways to reduce your stress level as you deal with the nursing home decision. Start here—

* if you are considering providing home care for your elderly parent and want to explore the pros and cons of that decision

* if you and your siblings or other close family members are in disagreement about how your parent should best be cared for

* if you are feeling any negative emotions, such as anxiety or guilt, about your parent's situation or about the long-term-care decision

* if your parent is in a nursing home now but tries hard to make you feel bad about it

* if you want to be supportive of a friend or loved one who is going through the process of making the nursing home decision

* if you are simply unsure what to do about your parent's or other loved one's current situation

* if the very idea of a nursing home makes you shudder

Part II, "You've Decided ... Now What?" discusses what to do once you've made the decision to get professional long-term care. It will help you determine which type of long-term-care facility is best for you and your loved one. It also discusses how to find and choose a quality facility. This is where you will find detailed descriptions of the various kinds of long-term-care facilities. Part II also offers strategies for making the transition into long-term care smoother and easier for everyone concerned. Start here—

* if you have decided to move your parent or loved one into a long-term-care facility, but don't yet know what type is right for him or her

* if you know what kind of facility your parent needs but haven't chosen a specific one

* if you have chosen a nursing home for your parent and want to know if you've made the right choice

* if you have chosen a nursing home for your parent but haven't moved him or her in yet

* if you have moved your parent into a nursing home and are wondering how he or she will adjust

Part III, "Making the Most of Life in a Nursing Home," will show you how to optimize life in a long-term-care institution, whether for yourself or for a family member. You can go right to this part of the book—

* if your parent is already living in a nursing home and you (and the other people involved) feel fine about that choice

* if you need reassurance and information about what nursing homes are really like on the inside

* if your parent is already living in a nursing home and you want to know how to be more involved in his or her life

* if your parent is already living in a nursing home but you or your parent has some complaints about the facility

* if your parent is living in a nursing home and you aren't genuinely enjoying your visits together

* if your parent is living in a nursing home and you want to get a sense of what his or her day-to-day life is like

Many points in this book are illustrated with real-life stories taken from our professional experiences and personal lives. Some of the stories come from nursing homes owned by Xenia; others took place in other long-term-care facilities. To protect their privacy, the names of all the people in the stories have been changed, and some of the individuals portrayed are composites of more than one person. Likewise, the fictionally named Mountain View Nursing Home is a composite of several nursing homes. We hope you will see similarities to your own situation in some of the stories and examples, and that you will find hope, reassurance, and value in them.

A number of exercises, worksheets, and checklists are included throughout the book to assist you with the processes of discovery, planning, and navigating the nursing home decision. Use the ones that feel appropriate to your situation. Take time to reflect on the questions before you answer them. Doing so can allow you to move through this challenging experience more easily and to make your decisions with confidence and clarity.

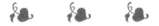

In her professional career and personal travels, Xenia has been inside nursing homes and talked with long-term-care professionals across the United States and in Europe. Regardless of where our elders are being cared for, the concerns are the same. If you are a nursing home resident, you want to feel safe, comfortable, respected, cared for, and "at home" in your facility. If you are a nursing home staff member, you want to feel good about what you do for a living and about the contribution you are making to people's lives. If you are a nursing home director, you want a facility that runs smoothly, where the staff enjoys working, the residents enjoy living, and everyone's needs are being met. And if you are the family member of a nursing home resident, you want to feel good about your loved one's care. You want to trust the facility, you want to know you made the best decision possible, you want to be confident about how your parent is being cared for, and you want to believe that your parent is happy (at least as happy as your particular parent is likely to be able to be).

It is our sincere hope that by the time you finish reading this book, you will know without a doubt that you have done the best you can do.

Chapter 1

Stepping into New Territory

John and Martha had been married for more than fifty years. They still lived in the same house where they had raised their two children. Their son, John Jr., served in the military overseas. Their daughter, Catherine, lived about an hour away with her husband and two young children.

For over twenty years John had suffered from Parkinson's disease. What began as occasional minor episodes of stiffness and trembling had gradually progressed to serious attacks, rendering him more and more helpless. John had always been an athletic, outdoorsy man, and he hated the idea of being sick. He had long ago decided that nobody would ever know about his problems. The disease was his and Martha's "little secret," and Martha simply took over caring for him whenever he needed extra help.

At first Martha enjoyed her new role. It made her feel powerful, needed, and important. But as John grew more helpless and less communicative, she began to resent his sickness and the toll it was taking on her body and mind. Martha wasn't getting any younger, and she was often exhausted from caring for John and managing the household without any help. Sometimes she scolded John, cursed his stiff muscles, or even accused him of not "cooperating" when she found it particularly difficult to dress or clean him.

Keeping John's condition a secret worked fine until the day Martha fell and broke her hip. She lay whimpering on the floor, and John could do nothing to help her. He simply sat and stared at his wife until she passed out from the pain. Several hours later, on the other side of town, Catherine, John and Martha's daughter, was outside raking leaves when her phone rang. She was shocked to learn that her mother was in the hospital and had just come out of hip surgery. Her father was there too, but couldn't be sent home by himself. Could she come immediately?

As she jumped into her car and headed for the hospital, Catherine felt baffled. She had spoken to her mother on the phone just that morning, and Martha had assured her that everything was fine. Whenever Catherine had asked about Dad over the years, Martha had reassured her that he was "just getting older, that's all." Although she had long suspected something wasn't quite right, Catherine never imagined the full extent of her father's condition or her mother's responsibilities. Now, out of the blue, these had suddenly become her responsibilities, and she had no idea what she was supposed to do.

Catherine, John, and Martha are real people with a real problem. We have changed their names, but their story is true and could be similar to yours. Like Catherine, you may have been taken completely by surprise by your parent's need for intervention and care. Or perhaps you knew it was coming, and now it has. What is the first thing you need to know? Here it is:

You can get through this and you will

We'll revisit Catherine later to see how her situation with John and Martha unfolds. For now, just know that you are not alone. If you are responsible for the well-being of a parent or another loved one, whether you came by that responsibility suddenly or gradually, know that there are millions of other people in the same situation. In North America and Europe, more than half a million residents will enter a nursing home for the first time this year. In the United States alone, 257,000 residents went into nursing homes last year.

Why We Feel So Bad about Nursing Homes

Most of us have heard negative things about nursing homes. From what we've observed, there is almost a knee-jerk reaction against the idea of being "put into" a nursing home. In many people's minds, a "good" son or daughter would never do such a thing to his or her mother or father. The very idea often brings up issues of abandonment and feelings of guilt, anger, hostility, and betrayal.

Why do we hear so many awful things about nursing homes? We believe there are both internal and external answers to this question. The biggest internal reason is the fact that none of us like to think about aging or death. Nursing homes are constant reminders of both. When we see our loved ones needing care, we can't help but realize on some level that one day we will very likely need the same kind of care ourselves. We don't like to think about this, so we blame the nursing homes for reminding us of our own vulnerabilities.

Among the external reasons why we hear bad things about nursing homes is because "nursing home" is an umbrella term that covers many different facilities and even *types* of facilities (see the next section, "What We Mean When We Say 'Nursing Home' "), some of which have real problems when it comes to care and funding and others which deal with resident populations that are difficult to provide care for. However, media bias also colors our view. The major media—radio, television, and print—are in business to make money. They are experts at discovering what sells and, simply put, negativity sells. People tend to be drawn to the dark side of things. This is why you will never turn on your television news program and hear how many thousands or even millions of people made it home safely last night. You *will* hear about the two or three who didn't—because this is the kind of news that gets people hooked. It is also part of what leads many people to develop a skewed and fearful view of life in general.

When was the last time you saw a news story about the active social communities, friendships, or even romances that develop in nursing homes? When did you last read something positive about the creative, patient, and dedicated people who care for our elders day in and day out? We make the mistake of thinking that because we don't hear about the positive aspects of nursing homes, they don't exist. Just like the people who make it home safely every night, in the world of nursing homes many people have positive and satisfying experiences. We share some of their stories with you in this book.

Another reason why nursing homes are easy targets of criticism is because a nursing home is an institution, while the victim of harm, when there is one, is always an individual. Whenever we hear stories of an individual versus an institution, we almost automatically identify with the individual. The institution becomes the "bad guy." The truth is that nursing homes are busy, active communities populated with real people, some of whom live there and some of whom work there. They interact with each other every day in close and personal ways, and, just like in "real" life outside the nursing home, sometimes there are problems between two or more of them. That's how life is. Unfortunately, if one of the people accused of wrongdoing happens to be a staff member of a nursing home, the story is usually reported as though the home itself were the culprit, which can make nursing homes in general seem like scary places indeed.

We're not saying that all nursing homes are created equal or that a nursing home should always be your first choice, but for some people, making the move to a long-term-care facility can be the very *best* option. For Mary-Ellen McKay it presented a whole new beginning.

> Eighty-two-year-old Mary-Ellen lived alone in a third-floor Santa Monica walk-up apartment she had shared with her late husband. Her only visitor was a friend who stopped by once a week. The two women had worked together as physician's assistants some twenty years earlier. Mary-Ellen's children all lived busy lives of their own, and though they called frequently, they were much too far away to look after their mother.

The stairs leading up to Mary-Ellen's apartment were difficult to manage, so she rarely went out except for an occasional walk to the corner market to pick up a few necessities. After a while even this became too challenging, so she stopped going out. Then she started falling down.

It was clear that Mary-Ellen needed help. Her friend encouraged her to move into a quality nursing home nearby. Once she did, her life changed dramatically for the better. First, the facility's doctor evaluated her medications. He determined that she was severely overmedicated and vulnerable to some potentially dangerous drug interactions. As soon as her medications were changed, Mary-Ellen showed a renewed interest in what was happening around her. She perked up, stopped falling, and started participating in the facility's community activities. She now has a boyfriend, several confidantes among the other residents, and an immense enjoyment of life. Her newfound happiness and improved health would never have been possible had she stayed isolated in her lonely apartment.

What We Mean When We Say "Nursing Home"

Before we go any further we want to clarify some terminology. Throughout this book we tend to use the phrases "nursing home" and "long-term-care facility" interchangeably. We do this only for convenience. There are differences. "Long-term care" (or "LTC") is an umbrella term that applies to any kind of care that someone receives on an ongoing basis. It may include long-term care at home, or more commonly, at the various kinds of facilities we refer to in this book. Some examples of long-term-care facilities are the following:

* Assisted-living centers
* Nursing homes or skilled nursing centers
* Convalescent homes

* Board-and-care facilities

* Retirement facilities

* Alzheimer's or memory-impairment facilities

In Chapter 6 we describe these various types of residential pro-grams in detail, with a specific focus on those that care for people who really can't live alone any longer (for whatever reason). In the book's title we use the phrase "nursing home" because it is the term most people are familiar with, but it will be up to you, using the information you find in these pages, to determine what type of facility is right for yourself or your loved one.

What We Mean When We Say "You"

Throughout this book we speak to you, the reader, in two senses of the word "you." We speak to you as the adult child of an elderly parent (or as the person responsible for the well-being of another elderly loved one) who needs your help and assistance. We also speak to you if you are trying to make the long-term-care decision for yourself. As we said in the Introduction, even though through-out the book we refer to the nursing home resident as "your par-ent," this book isn't just about parents.

We are aware that many potential long-term-care residents are perfectly capable of evaluating their choices and making decisions for themselves. If this describes you, you may be tired of doing your own housekeeping, or you may need a little help getting dressed in the morning, but you are still of sound mind and are just exploring your options. This book is for you whether you are considering making the move to live with one of your children or whether you simply want to know more about long-term-care facilities. It is also for you if you are already a resident of a long-term-care facility and want to know how to make your stay more satisfying and pleasant. Although this book is written as though it is addressed to the adult sons or daughters of elderly people, all the information in it can be applied to oneself as well.

We are also aware that readers will come to this book at many different stages in the process of either making the nursing home decision or learning how to live well in a nursing home. If you haven't done so already, please review the section in the Introduction titled "How to Read This Book" to help you determine where in the book you can find information addressed to your particular circumstances.

Some Assumptions

This book was written with two simple assumptions in mind that you'll need to know to get the most out of reading it. The first assumption we make is that each person is responsible for his or her own level of happiness and satisfaction. We may not be able to fully control our life circumstances, but we can control our reactions to those circumstances. You are not responsible for your parents' happiness any more than your parents are responsible for yours. You may be able to help your parents cope with their circumstances, but you are not responsible for their situation.

We know this is not as simple as it sounds, so we spend plenty of time in Chapter 5 exploring the various feelings that arise when the nursing home decision becomes a necessity. Don't worry if you're not fond of or familiar with working things out on the emotional level. We provide a simple primer that anyone can use to learn more about emotions in general and also about what to do with uncomfortable feelings when they pop up.

The second assumption we make is that in a relationship with your parent you would prefer to be a "love-giver" rather than just a caregiver. A caregiver is someone who attends to another person's survival and physical comfort needs. Caregiving can be an act of love, but it is not about the relationship between the caregiver and the care recipient. A love-giver attends to the emotional and relationship needs of another person. The two roles are not mutually exclusive, but all too often people exhaust themselves and their resources (emotional and physical) providing basic care and, as a result, have nothing left for the important and rewarding tasks of maintaining a loving and fulfilling relationship. If you have to spend all your time feeding, washing, and assisting your parent at the expense of your own interests and self-care, it can be very difficult to also enjoy a satisfying relationship with him or her. In this book, we assume that, whenever possible, it is better to delegate the caregiving role and to use one's limited life energy to fill the love-giving role.

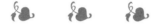

When an elderly loved one needs your help over the long haul, there is a lot to think about. You may feel the instinctive desire to bring her or him home to live with you. Or maybe you feel pressure to do that from within yourself or from outside sources, such as your siblings, other relatives, or even your parents themselves. You may be resigned to having to put your mother or father into a nursing home, but you don't feel very good about it and don't know quite where to start.

If you are in a situation where you need to make decisions about the care of an elderly loved one, you've come to the right place. In the chapters that follow, we'll walk you through the decision process step-by-step and point out the most important things for you to consider at each stage along the way. We'll assuage your fears and doubts and help you make the most of your remaining time with your loved one. As we've pointed out before, you can get through this and you will. Follow the advice in this book and you'll be able to make your elder-care decisions with the confidence that comes from being fully informed.

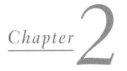

The Phone Call That Will Change Your Life

To everything there is a season, and a time to every
purpose under heaven.

— *Ecclesiastes 3:1*

Beth stood in the middle of her garden, took a look around, and smiled. She had been devoted to her family for the past twenty years. Now that her youngest child had left for college, it was finally her turn. She looked forward to indulging her lifelong passion for gardening and even planned to start a new career. As Beth pulled weeds she daydreamed about teaching gardening to local schoolchildren and perhaps even hosting a gardening show on a local television station. She breathed in deeply, smelled the freshly turned earth, and smiled again. Life didn't get any better than this.

Beth's mobile phone roused her. It was her older brother, Jack, a busy tax attorney. "Mom's had a stroke," he cried. "She's in the hospital. It's really serious." In that instant Beth stopped daydreaming. She knew exactly what she had to do. She wanted her mother, Gwen, to survive. She knew she would take care of her, and this would mean bringing her mother home to live with her. As she pulled off her garden boots and ran inside the house, Beth looked around her place with fresh eyes. She thought about where an old and sick person might be comfortable. She imagined her mother sitting in a wheelchair before the fireplace or at the window looking out into Beth's beautiful garden. She pictured Gwen smiling with gratitude for all Beth was doing for her.

When Beth phoned her husband at his office, he, too, was shocked by the news of Gwen's stroke—but for a different reason. He had never really appreciated his mother-in-law. Over the years, just to keep the peace, he had learned to withdraw a bit and bite his tongue when he was around her. Those moments together had been few, so he had simply shrugged off the relationship. But now she would be coming to live with them....

You may know someone a bit like Beth. Just as her life appeared to be her own for the first time in years, her mother's stroke changed everything. A phone call changed her life.

One day, you may get a similar call. If your parents are still alive, which nowadays they are likely to be, the odds are good that you will receive an unsettling phone call about one of them when you are in middle age. You may have anticipated the call for months, or you may be surprised. You may have dreaded it, or you may have dismissed it as one of those things that happen to other people but not to you. When you get the call, you will pick up the phone and hear that something has happened to your mother or father or another loved one, that he or she is helpless and needs you, if not immediately then very soon, perhaps in a few days, after being released from the hospital. When this happens, you will have to drop whatever you are doing, turn off the stove, end the phone call, cancel the meeting, and get to where your parent is from wherever you are.

You may have already received that call, or you may have known for some time that your loved one is suffering from Alzheimer's disease or Parkinson's disease or some other degenerative condition that will require you to intervene in his or her life sooner or later. Perhaps this time has come, and you may be asking yourself, "Now what?"

Here Come the Changes!

Suddenly (or perhaps not so suddenly), you find yourself faced with the awareness that you are supposed to change your schedule, change your family life, change your professional goals, and change your personal interests. You must completely change your life so you can take responsibility for the person who gave it to you in the first place. How do you do it? What is the best course of action? What is the "right" thing to do?

You have been pulled into a problem made more complex by vast historic, economic, and medical changes (more on that in the next chapter), and now you are being forced to make some changes yourself. Don't worry. Changes like this can be daunting and confusing, but after reading this chapter you'll know more about what to expect, and you'll be able to make plans and decisions more easily. Once you understand the factors behind the decisions you're faced with and have fully explored the alternatives, you will be more confident about your choices regarding your parents' care.

In this chapter you will learn some basic information about how change can affect your life and what you can do to deal with it. You'll learn about managing change-related stress, and you'll determine your own stress level by working through the exercise at the end of the chapter.

Making Friends with Change

Change is a constant force in our lives, and these days it seems to occur faster all the time. We are continuously bombarded with new information, new inventions, and new situations. You may think that with all this steady change happening we would simply relax and get used to it, but that's easier said than done. Letting go is scary. Change, whether positive or negative, is almost always stressful, and extreme change can make us feel overwhelmed and out of control. Whether control is real or only an illusion, we all like to feel in control of as many aspects of our lives as we can. It makes us feel safer to think that we are able to predict and prepare for events.

Several factors affect how much stress we experience when faced with a change, including—

* whether the change was expected or whether it came as a surprise
* whether the change is viewed as "good" or "bad"
* how far-reaching the effects of the change are in our lives
* how much control we have in the face of the change
* how much support we have to help us cope with the change
* how well we understand the reasons behind the change

Let's take a deeper look at these issues.

WAS THE CHANGE A SURPRISE OR WAS IT EXPECTED?

Saul, eighty-two, realized that his heart condition would probably allow him to live only a few more years. He also saw that his wife, Rachel, was beginning to lose her short-term memory. So Saul asked his two grown children, Aaron and Deborah, to pay him a visit. When they arrived, Saul told them that he planned to transfer all his assets into a trust for the care of their mother. The two children would be equally responsible trustees. After Saul's death, they would use the money to care for their mother until she died, at which time the remaining assets would be shared equally between them.

Saul's advance planning and open communication paid off. When he died two years later, Aaron and Deborah knew exactly what to do. By that time their mother's short-term memory had deteriorated to the point where she could no longer live alone. Aaron and Deborah, who lived in different states, used the trust to hire and pay for a caregiver to visit Rachel daily. As Rachel's dementia advanced, more caregivers were hired, until she had around-the-clock care in her own home. Once it was clear that Rachel no longer knew where she was, Aaron moved her into a fine nursing home near where he lived. He was able to visit her daily until she died some years later.

It is certainly easier to deal with change that we have been expecting for a while. Of course, not all parents are as forthcoming with their health and financial information as Saul was with Aaron and Deborah, but Saul's decision made the inevitable change much easier for everyone involved. It still wasn't "easy" for Aaron and Deborah. They still lost their father, and even though they knew it was coming they still went through a normal grieving period. And in a way, they lost their mother, too, long before she actually died, and that was hard. But Saul helped Aaron and Deborah anticipate the changes that he could help them with, and his doing so made things easier for them.

When change happens unexpectedly, it can be much harder to deal with. We must make decisions quickly, and we don't always have all the information we need to make them well. It isn't always clear what our best course of action should be. It isn't always clear what our parents want (or would have wanted). And even if we know their wishes, it isn't always clear that what they want is really in their own best interests.

Suddenly, in the course of one unexpected phone call, we may be thrust into the role of being a parent to someone who once parented us. A dramatic change is triggered that touches us on all levels: physical, mental, emotional, and spiritual. Suddenly we have to consider what it means to "honor thy father and mother," as so many of us were raised to do. Does "to honor" mean to do whatever they wish, even when their mental faculties are fading? Or does it mean to do what we believe in our heart is best for them, even if they don't like it? How to best care for our parents when the need is sudden is a very personal and very difficult decision. It is one that our friend Amy faced recently.

Late one rainy night, Amy received a call from a hostile-sounding stranger who identified himself as a police officer. He said, "You should take better care of your mother!"

Amy, shocked, had no idea what he was talking about. Her widowed mother, Ruth, lived about an hour away. Although they hadn't seen each other since last Thanksgiving, they spoke often by phone and had a good relationship. In fact, Amy had spoken to Ruth that afternoon, and everything had seemed fine.

Several minutes and many questions later, Amy was able to determine that her mother, wearing only a nightgown, had wandered out of her house at 10:00 P.M., to "go shopping." When the police picked Ruth up in an intersection, she was soaked, confused, and disoriented. When they asked her where she lived, she grew belligerent and wouldn't tell them. They took her to the station and found her I.D. in her handbag. A neighbor gave them Amy's phone number.

Amy and her husband, Mike, rushed to the police station. When they arrived, they found Ruth wrapped in a blanket. Amy felt guilty that she hadn't thought to bring any dry clothes with her. Ruth was extremely upset and agitated. "She told us the police had taken away all her clothes and were making her sit there in her pajamas," Amy says, shaking her head. "She even threatened to sue them!"

When Amy gently suggested that her mother come home with them, Ruth grew hostile and angry. "I know my rights!" she yelled. "You're still my child and I'm still your mother. You take me to my house this instant!" Amy and Mike looked at each other. There didn't seem to be anything else they could do but what Ruth was ordering them to do. So they took Ruth to her house. When they got there it was nearly 2:00 in the morning. The front door stood wide open. Ruth had simply walked out of the house without locking up. Everything was okay inside the house, but what would happen tomorrow or the next day?

Ruth angrily insisted that Amy and Mike leave her alone and get out of her house. Not knowing what else to do, they drove home. The next morning, when Amy spoke with her mother on the phone, Ruth was back to her old self. She seemed not to remember the incident at all, and when Amy mentioned it Ruth suggested that Amy was losing her mind and might want to consider seeing a psychiatrist.

Her new living arrangement was stressful and challenging at times. She missed her friends from the old neighborhood, and she got a bit "stir crazy" during the winter months, but by viewing her change as a positive one overall, Julia made it easier on herself and on her children. Her children benefit now by knowing that their mother is part of a community that cares for her. They will also benefit in the future. When Julia dies, her children will not be left having to determine how to dispose of her home and possessions, or wondering what her wishes would be. Julia has taken care of all of that for them.

Everyone in Julia's family views the change in her life as a good one. There were some stresses and it was a big job, but overall the change went smoothly. It would have been far more difficult if one of her children had decided it was bad for Julia to move out of her home. If Julia had believed the move was a bad idea, she never would have made it and would probably have stayed isolated in her home. She eventually would have found it increasingly difficult to get out and about. At that point her children would have had far more dramatic and unpleasant changes to deal with.

When the phone call about your parent comes, no matter how unexpected or traumatic the change that ensues, you can make it easier on yourself by trying not to judge it as a bad thing. Perhaps you won't be able to go so far as to view your parent's challenges as a good thing. That's understandable. But if you can see them as neutral—as a "this is just how things are" situation—you'll help to make the changes much easier for yourself and everyone around you to deal with.

HOW FAR-REACHING ARE THE EFFECTS OF THE CHANGE?

One reason it was easy for Julia's children to accept her decision to move into a retirement home was because the changes didn't affect them very much. They faced some small changes, like contacting her at a different address, calling her at a different phone number, and flying to a different airport when visiting her, but none of those changes had a major impact on their lives. Contrast this with Bert's situation:

Bert, a fifty-five-year-old doctor in a small town, was in his office when he received a phone call from the hospital. He was used to getting calls from the hospital about his patients, but this one was different. It was about his father, Albert.

Albert, age seventy-three, had fallen from his favorite stool in the local bar and hurt himself. Bert asked a lot of questions. He learned that Albert was suffering from advanced cirrhosis of the liver. His abdomen was swollen, and his arms and legs were very thin because the muscles had wasted away. He exhibited symptoms of Korsakow syndrome, a serious and irreversible brain disorder caused by years of heavy drinking.

Bert knew his father would not live much longer. It might be a few weeks or several months before he died, but Albert would be unable to live on his own when he was released from the hospital. Bert was accustomed to dealing with sick and dying people, but this time it was personal—and far more complicated than treating an ordinary patient. Bert and Albert had not spoken in five years, since Bert's wedding to his second wife, Susan. At the reception Albert had gotten drunk and said some things that left Susan in tears. Such behavior had been typical of Albert for as long as Bert could remember. His father could not keep promises and was totally out of control after a few drinks. Albert was such a heavy drinker that Bert thought it was a miracle his father had lived so long.

After he hung up the phone, Bert reflected on his difficult childhood. The family was always moving from one run-down apartment to another, chased by unpaid debts. Bert, the eldest of five children, had worked to help support the family since early childhood. Somewhere along the way he had learned to hate his father. He was struck with the realization that this was his last chance to learn something more about Albert. He wanted to hear about his father's life, his fears and dreams, and maybe even learn a thing or two about himself. Bert decided to bring his father home from the hospital and to spend Albert's last days caring for him and healing their relationship.

As a doctor, Bert has some idea of what he is getting into in caring for Albert's physical needs. But he has no idea how much change is about to hit him on the emotional and mental levels, areas that he's neglected for many years. Bert's decision will have profound effects not only on his own life but also on those of Albert and of Susan, Bert's wife. Bert is taking on these challenges voluntarily, but without a full awareness of their impact.

We'll revisit Bert and Albert in a later chapter. At this point it is important for you to know one thing. If you're faced with making a decision about caring for your elderly parents, be sure to consider the full impact it will have on your life and on the lives of those around you. Will the change mostly affect only your parent? Or only you and your parent? Or will it also affect your spouse, your children, your siblings, and possibly even your neighbors? Will the changes be small, such as occasionally visiting a nursing home? Or will they be larger, such as rearranging your schedule and home life so you can take on the care of your parent yourself? Will you have to dispose of your parent's home and possessions? If so, is the home nearby? Will you have any help from your siblings?

It may seem difficult at this moment to determine what the effects of such a decision can be. Hang in there and keep reading. One of the aims of this book is to give you a better idea of the areas in your life that will be impacted by whatever choice you make. We hope to help you decide with much more confidence whether you are doing the right thing for yourself and your loved ones. For now, just know that the more extensive the effects of any change are, the more stressful they will be to cope with.

HOW MUCH CONTROL DO YOU HAVE?

Another factor that influences how well we deal with change is the amount of control we believe we have. In the case of Saul, who took care of his finances when he was still able to do so, his children felt more in control and less stressed than they would have otherwise. In the case of Amy, whose mother, Ruth, wanders around at night but refuses to admit that anything is wrong, Amy has no control and therefore experiences a great deal of stress.

If you have no idea what goes on in a nursing home, you will feel uneasy about your ability to control and influence your parent's life. We think this book, especially the stories in Part III about life inside a nursing home, will give you a feel for what really happens in long-term-care facilities. Having this knowledge will help you decide confidently whether a nursing home is right for your loved one.

HOW MUCH SUPPORT DO YOU HAVE?

Support can be thought of as the flip side of control. If you have complete control of a situation, it's usually because you're the only one calling all the shots. This can be efficient and less stressful than having to negotiate with someone else at every step along the way, but it can also mean you may be low on support. Good support can make all the difference in how well we cope with difficult changes. When your parents need your help, support can come from your siblings, your spouse, your spiritual counselor, your friends and neighbors, your therapist, hired caregivers, and possibly even organizations set up to deal with your situation. Support also comes in many forms, including words of appreciation and praise. Remember to ask for the kind of support you need.

Of course, support can have a dark side. If five siblings disagree about how an elderly parent should be cared for, things can get more stressful than ever. If this is the case in your family, be sure that everyone involved has a chance to express his or her thoughts and to be fully heard. Discussions of parental care can be dangerous ground and, if handled insensitively, can irreparably damage relationships. But they can also provide an opportunity for siblings to bond at a more intimate level if everyone feels that he or she is being heard and that his or her feelings are being respected.

When it comes to caring for a parent, emotions often get in the way of clear conversation, creating a scenario that can drain a lot of energy from everyone involved. Never argue with a sibling or parent about choices and decisions that need to be made. When you argue with someone, you force that person to defend him- or herself, and the only way most people know how to do this is to argue back or grow even more uncooperative. It may take longer to reach a decision when differing opinions are involved, but building a consensus will ensure you of the best possible support from your family. Make sure everyone in the group knows how everyone else feels, and then, if possible, come to a compromise that everyone can agree to live with. If tensions are running high in your family, see the advice and exercise in Chapter 10 about resolving conflicts between family members.

HOW WELL IS THE CHANGE UNDERSTOOD?

We generally cope better with a change if we understand the reasons behind it than we do if the change seems random. Change that we perceive as random makes us feel unsafe and perhaps worried that something terrible may happen. So we try hard to explain changes to ourselves. When we have an explanation for a given change, we can usually cope with it much more effectively. For example, many of the health and even behavioral problems our parents may experience can be explained as normal consequences of aging. When we know and accept this, we can at least feel a little better. The problems our parents are facing are not likely to strike us too—at least not until we are closer to their ages.

Exercise: Determining Your Personal Change-Related Stress Level

We have discussed some of the factors that can make change easier or more difficult to deal with. This quiz can help you gauge the amount of stress you're experiencing in relation to the specific changes you're going through right now. For each numbered item, simply circle the answer that best describes your current situation with your parents. Remember that there are no right or wrong answers; the purpose is simply to get a better understanding of how much stress you are under at the moment. Sometimes this alone can make you feel better.

1. When I found out I had to make decisions about my parent's care
   a. I knew this time was coming and was as prepared as I could be.
   b. I suspected this time was coming, but I wasn't really prepared.
   c. I was taken completely by surprise.

2. What has happened in our family regarding my parent(s) is
   a. a terrific development. I'll be able to sleep much better now.
   b. a normal consequence of aging. We'll deal with it okay.
   c. a terribly difficult thing that I wouldn't want anyone else to have to go through.

3. The decision I am leaning toward making will
   a. mostly affect only my parent.
   b. mostly just affect my parent and me.
   c. affect not just my parent and me, but other family members as well, such as my spouse, children, and siblings.

4. The decision I am leaning toward making will be
   a. pretty easy to manage.
   b. a bit challenging at first. There will be assets to be disposed of and other things to deal with. But after that, things will be easier.
   c. a big change for all of us. It may include changing my schedule, my lifestyle, and/or the interior of my home.

5. The degree of control I have over this change is
   a. a good amount. It's all in my hands, or if not, the person(s) I am sharing the decision with and I agree on just about everything.

    b. a reasonable amount. I'm not 100 percent in charge, and things don't always go my way, but I feel that my contribution has an impact and is of some value.

    c. none! I can't make any difference in the situation at this time.

6. At this point in my life

    a. I have adequate time and resources (money, insurance, assistance, etc.) to devote to making this decision on behalf of my parent.

    b. I am juggling several other responsibilities or struggling with coming up with enough resources to handle this decision.

    c. I have no time to deal with this situation, and/or I do not have adequate resources available to me in this situation.

7. In terms of support

    a. I feel I have exactly what I need to get through this.

    b. I could use a little more support from someone—maybe more than one person.

    c. I feel completely unsupported. I need much more help than I am currently receiving.

Look back over your answers and count how many a's, b's, and c's you've circled. Write down your total for each:

_____ a's   _____ b's   _____ c's

Mostly a's: You are in good shape. You're facing changes and challenges, but they are unlikely to be exceedingly difficult for you. Continue reading this book to gain more clarity, insight, and ideas about what to expect, but you should do just fine in the stress department.

Some or mostly b's: You are facing a bit more stress in dealing with your situation than may be healthy for you and your loved ones. See if there are any areas that you can convert to a's. Reconsider any decision you are making that causes you more stress than necessary. Ask for (or hire) help when you need it. And please keep reading. The information contained in this book can offer guidance in how to do all of these things.

Some or mostly c's: You are under tremendous amounts of change-related stress. See if you can get some outside help in dealing with your situation. Therapists, assistants, and caregivers (either part-time or full-time) can all provide tremendous relief. Reevaluate any decisions you've made that are causing you and those you love any great upheaval. And finally, try your best to accept the things you cannot change. Some things just are. In those cases, your only choice lies in how you go about dealing with them. This book is designed to equip you to deal with them in the most beneficial way possible.

Equally important, be sure to take care of yourself. Exercise, get enough rest, drink plenty of water, and be sure to give yourself some daily quiet time. It may seem selfish to take care of your own needs first when someone else needs you so much, but if you don't, you will be unable to care for anyone else for very long. If you let your own health go, you will be the one needing care, and then the situation will grow even more complicated!

As we mentioned in the chapter's opening, you are not alone in your problems relating to change. Larger societal forces, especially those occurring in the last century, have impacted the aging process for everyone. Some of your feelings of responsibility, guilt, anxiety, or uncertainty may make much more sense in the context of the bigger picture. In the next chapter, we take a look at some of the large-scale changes that affect us all.

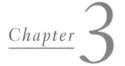

Chapter **3**

It's Bigger than We Are: Changes in Society That Have Affected Aging and Culture

When you learn that one of your parents needs your help, you may feel overwhelmed and isolated. Whom can you turn to for help and advice? Where are the answers? As difficult as your situation is, it is important to realize that you are not alone. Millions of other people and families are dealing with the same circumstances at this very moment.

If so many people are facing the same thing, why does the situation feel new and strange? Why can't we simply do what we have always done? The answer is that this situation *is* new and strange, for all of us. Our society has changed rapidly over the last several decades, and for the first time ever, elder-care is a widespread challenge.

Why Things Are Different for Our Generation

There are a number of reasons why we are among the first generation of people to face en masse the problem of aging parents. Let's take a look at some of them.

PEOPLE LIVE LONGER

People typically live longer now than they did only a generation or two ago. To put it bluntly, 150 years ago people did not have to worry as much about caring for elderly parents because their parents did not live anywhere near as long as people live today. In fact, only 100 years ago you yourself would probably not have lived as long as you already have. As Robert N. Butler, M.D., president of the International Longevity Center and professor of geriatrics at the Mount Sinai Medical Center, writes in a foreword to the *Consumer Reports Complete Guide for Health Services for Seniors*, "In 1900, the life span for most Americans was forty-seven," but by 1999, "a full 80 percent of all deaths occurred after age sixty-five." There are many reasons for this change, most of them related to modern medicine. Here's a list of some of the most important ones:

* Infant mortality rates have dropped dramatically; many more of us now survive birth and infancy.

* We have eliminated the most deadly childhood diseases of the past, such as polio and smallpox; many more of us now survive childhood.

* We have dramatically reduced the number of women's deaths during childbirth; many more of us now survive pregnancy.

* Diagnosis and treatment have been improved for chronic conditions such as kidney disease, diabetes, and hypertension, all of which used to kill large numbers of people; many more of us now survive into old age.

* The poorest people used to simply starve to death, but government-sponsored nutrition and health-care programs are now available to assist them; many more of us now survive poverty.

Diphtheria, pneumonia, smallpox, accidents, hunger, poor nutrition, tuberculosis, infections, polio, and chronic diseases like diabetes used to cause death at a relatively young age, even until fairly recently. All are commonly survived today. According to a 1998 publication from the U.S. Census Bureau, in 1850 the median age in the United States was 18.3—that is, half the population was under age 18.3 and half was over that age. This means a majority of people died before age 20. At the beginning of the twentieth century only about 3 percent of the U.S. population was older than 60. Life in those days was hard and conditions were often miserable. People aged much faster and died much younger, without any special nursing or medical treatment and without a sense of having any "good old days" to look back upon.

Compared to our great-grandparents, we're not just surviving; we're thriving. Less than two generations ago, something as simple as a broken leg that was not professionally set could mean a lifelong handicap, rendering one a cripple. That meant being unable to work as hard as others, being unable to earn a living, being unable to feed a family—in essence, being unable to survive. As much as we like to romanticize the past, our forebears enjoyed few "good old days."

PEOPLE LIVE A *LOT* LONGER!

Modern medicine no longer just saves lives; it can actually prolong life for decades beyond what was possible in previous generations. In fact, medical advances have added far more years to the average lifespan than anyone realized would ever be achievable. Recent medical discoveries and developments allow us to treat many diseases that were typically fatal to older and weaker people even just a few decades ago. For example, pneumonia was and is considered a serious and dangerous disease, but in most cases today it can be treated. According to the American Lung Association, until 1998 the number of deaths attributed to pneumonia increased annually to nearly a hundred thousand per year. Within one year, by 1999, that number had fallen (for the first time) to fewer than sixty-four thousand deaths, and it has continued to decrease every year since then.

Less than twenty years ago, a simple fall resulting in a broken hip was a death sentence for even the healthiest of older patients. It meant being immobilized in bed, suffering dramatic pain, and most likely experiencing pulmonary complications, which led to death after only a few weeks or months. The patient was unable to move or be moved or withstand even the lightest touch without suffering enormous pain. For someone in such a state, even a simple cold was often deadly. The patient could not cough because of the pain, so phlegm would settle in the lungs and promote the growth of bacteria. Pneumonia usually followed, and then death. Today, treatment of a hip fracture through the implantation of a new, artificial hip joint is a routine matter. Even the oldest patient can often expect to spend no more than ten days in the hospital, followed by some time in a rehab facility, with a good chance of ultimately returning to life as it was before the fracture.

Only ten years ago, it was considered unsafe to perform many surgical procedures on older patients. Today, medical progress has led to extremely refined methods of diagnosis, execution, and post-operative treatment, which make even high-risk surgeries acceptable for most older people.

EIGHTY IS THE NEW SIXTY: WE HAVE REDEFINED WHAT IT MEANS TO BE "OLD"

It would have been impossible for our great-grandparents to imagine living as long as the majority of people do today. As we've mentioned, "old" to our grandparents' generation usually meant fifty or sixty. Under the conditions of that era, a person was usually pretty worn out by that age. People in their late thirties often looked the way most sixty- or even seventy-year-olds do today.

A hundred years ago, having a body that was somehow wearing out meant becoming dependent and vulnerable and not having much of a quality of life at all. Nowadays, many nonfatal health problems that used to render people nearly helpless in their later years can be treated by routine interventions. Life for the elderly is now often a simple matter of compensating for certain weaknesses. For example, today we may think of a cataract as something easy to repair. Only twenty-five years ago, having a cataract meant being unable to take part in routine daily life. People with cataracts had to wear enormous glasses to be able to focus on a very small field; for everything else, they were nearly blind. Today, cataract repair is a routine outpatient procedure that many ophthalmologists perform right in their offices.

Other health issues that commonly crop up when people reach their fifties or sixties, like prostate problems or urinary incontinence, which used to lead to severe social challenges and daily inconvenience, can now be corrected by common medical treatment or surgery. Nowadays, forty-, fifty-, and even sixty-year-olds are considered to be in midlife. Many are beginning new careers or pursuing new passions. For the first time in history, these midlife people find themselves in the position of having to take care of their elderly parents.

THE POPULATION HAS AGED OVERALL

Today there are more older and fewer younger people alive than ever before. The U.S. Census Bureau has collected population statistics from nearly 250 countries and has projected the population trends until the year 2050. These data show that the societal changes discussed in this chapter have impacted countries around the world. In most Western (and many Eastern) countries, including the United States, members of the current oldest generation were born into families that had many children. The middle generation has its origins in families of two to four children. By contrast, the current young generation, the after-the-pill generation, typically has much smaller families. Today's more common one-child (or childless) family will be faced with accommodating and caring for the aging baby-boomer generation in less than three decades. In fact, according to the census data, the fastest-growing age group in the world population of people sixty-five and older is the group over age eighty-five!

If our parents had to care for their parents at all, they usually did so with the help of many more siblings (who lived much closer to each other) than we do today. And many of the older couples of tomorrow will not have any children at all. That means very soon fewer and fewer middle-aged people will be left to care for more and more elderly people.

FAMILIES ARE MORE MOBILE

Regardless of whether your origins are in a large wealthy farming family, a family of craftsmen, or a family in bondage or slavery, several generations ago your ancestors' extended family probably lived together in one village. In most cases they probably all lived in one house, and possibly they even lived in one room. All this changed as a result of one of the most important transformations ever to take place in human culture: the industrial revolution, which is widely considered to be one of the most significant nonmilitary revolutions in the history of the world. Once a society becomes industrialized its economy is no longer based on agriculture and craftsmanship but rather on production that takes place in large, mechanized plants and factories. In Europe and North America this change began occurring about two hundred years ago. For the first time, people had to "go to work." Within a few generations, children were no longer the measure of a family's wealth, but rather mouths that had to be fed. Families no longer had the farm to produce food for themselves; now they had to buy bread at the corner store. And the money needed to do so had to be earned somehow. Young people by the millions began leaving their parents and the countryside to find work in the cities.

Today, daily family life for the middle and younger generations is structured much differently from how it was even eighty years ago. Children commonly leave home by their late teens or early twenties to attend college or begin a career. Even before the children leave home for good, families are separated part of the time on most days. Both parents are likely to leave home each morning to go to work, and even small children frequently attend preschool or kindergarten. Nowadays, when young adults leave home to live on their own, their parents are likely to be somewhere between forty and sixty years old, healthy, vital, and full of plans for their future.

So are we midlifers a generation of "bad" children? Selfish individuals unwilling to think of our poor parents? Not at all. Today, both adult children and their parents enjoy being independent and living separate lives, while frequently enjoying warm relationships with each other, even if they're separated by miles. But we are experiencing a new challenge: Our parents, in a certain way, are "coming back." Over the last few decades, as young adults have grown up and moved out on their own, their parents have often left the traditional family home to create their own adventures. Maybe they enjoyed the warmth of the South or the fun of traveling through the country in a motor home. In most cases they didn't think much about needing care one day.

FAMILY STRUCTURES HAVE CHANGED

Not so long ago everyone in an extended family lived together and everyone pitched in. Work was a family affair and was not considered separate from everyday life. Today, not only are our work and home lives usually separate, at least to some degree, but our families look very different. High rates of divorce and remarriage have yielded large numbers of stepchildren, stepparents, and half siblings. It is not uncommon these days for children to be raised by four or even six parents, as their biological parents divorce and remarry multiple times.

Often, families that have regrouped over the years harbor deep (or not so deep) hostilities. Children don't always know their biological parents well and may feel closer to a stepparent. Half siblings may have as much to say about caring for an elderly parent as full siblings would. Today's family structures can make caring for our parents an even bigger challenge than anyone anticipated.

WOMEN'S ROLES HAVE CHANGED

Women are no longer the default caretakers in the home. In just the last fifteen to twenty years, more women have entered the workplace than ever before. According to the U.S. Census, between 1973 and 1993 the number of women over age twenty-five who were enrolled in college doubled. Now those college-educated women are far more likely to be involved in career work than in full-time housework. These days, a woman may interrupt her career to raise her children and provide a home life for her husband, but most women don't see themselves remaining in this type of caregiving role for the rest of their lives.

For several reasons, most women do not want to or cannot afford to give up their jobs to take over the full-time duties of in-home care for an elderly parent. Perhaps they are divorced and living on their own, or are single parents, or simply have to contribute to the family income to make ends meet. Whatever the reason, it can no longer be assumed that women will just be waiting at home to take care of someone who needs assistance.

Comparison: Then and Now

We have discussed a number of societal changes that directly impact the way we need to care for our parents. Here is a summary of some of these changes:

Society Yesterday and Today	
THEN	**NOW**
High infant-mortality rates	Low infant-mortality rates
High rate of death in childbirth	Mothers usually survive childbirth
Most people died before age 20	Most people live beyond age 60
Chronic diseases killed many	Many chronic diseases have been controlled
Harsh survival conditions	Conditions make it much easier to survive
40 and 50 considered old age	80 and 90 considered old age
Older people grew helpless	Many older people now enjoy vital lives
Large families (many children)	Smaller families (fewer children)
Families stayed close together	Families are spread out

Society Yesterday and Today (cont'd.)	
THEN	**NOW**
The population included very few older people	The population includes more older people than younger people
Families worked together	Family members have their own professions
Nuclear families stayed intact	Families split apart and reform
Women stayed home and were the caregivers	Women work outside the home

Past Ways of Caring

The problem of caring for the weaker and sicker members of society has always been with us. When your parent needs more care than you can provide, you may feel somehow inadequate, as though there is an existing standard somewhere out there that you are failing to live up to. If this is the case, you may feel better knowing a bit about the way care used to be provided and the way it can be provided now.

As recently as two and three generations ago, the mantra of the times could have been "Whoever doesn't work doesn't get fed." For most families, life was about basic survival, and there was little energy or time for anything more. In those days, the responsibilities of caring for the youngest children and for sick adults were often integrated into everyday life, without interrupting the necessary work. "Caring" was done with the least possible effort. Those who couldn't yet do or who no longer did "real" work, usually older children and older adults, had to take care of the others.

Until the turn of the twentieth century, the level of care provided to older or sick people was generally kept to a bare minimum, out of necessity. This care was viewed as a matter of charity rather than as a matter of true caring, knowledge, or expertise. It was nearly always a short-term endeavor, lasting only a few days, weeks, or maybe months, but rarely years. Back then, most major towns had a few charity institutions designed to care for the sick, especially those who were dying. These "poor houses" were places of extreme misery, nasty smells, and severe pain. Dozens of dying people might have been warehoused in one large room, living amid their own excrement and bleeding from wounds and sores. No wonder "putting someone in a home" has such terrible connotations. Most people probably would rather have died alone in the forest than be sent to live out their last days in such desolation.

As recently as our parents' generation, for the first time in history, older people often stayed back home in the country while the young ones moved to the cities in search of work. Often the elders who remained in the country were taken care of by neighbors or extended family members. In the last forty or fifty years, urban-dwelling older people who survived adulthood and whose kids had gone off to other places to find work began dying alone in their apartments, in hospitals, or in "rest homes."

BUT MY MOM TOOK CARE OF *HER* PARENTS!

On the other hand, only a generation or two ago, many mothers of young children who could afford to stay at home usually took over the care of older family members. Your own mother is very likely to have cared for her parents at home, which may have led her to expect the same from you. Perhaps you have even unconsciously internalized these expectations for yourself, without really having thought much about it. You may harbor these expectations even though today's circumstances are very different and your loved one's condition may not be conducive to home care. It is important to be aware of and to understand any such expectations you may be living with, as these are a frequent source of guilt and anxiety for children of older people.

Coping with Longevity

It may seem that living longer is always a good thing, but all this medical progress has created a new set of problems. Older people must contend with living in a fast-paced, busy culture that was not designed for those with weaknesses. Yes, people now survive to a ripe old age, but they usually need some support—often for many years. Older people's years-long need for support is very new to our culture. Fortunately, we're getting better and better at dealing with it. These days, the most common problems of old age can generally be compensated for in four major ways:

1. Through special/technical equipment

2. Through medication

3. With help/assistance

4. Through providing care

WE CAN PROVIDE BETTER EQUIPMENT THAN EVER BEFORE

Many of the current handicaps associated with aging can now be compensated for with special equipment:

* If we have poor vision, we can wear corrective lenses.

* If the stairs are too difficult, we can take the elevator or escalator.

* If we can't walk very far, we can drive (and perhaps park in a handicapped spot) or take a bus.

* If we can't carry our groceries, we can use a cart.

* If we have problems with hearing, we can get a hearing aid.

* If we have problems with balance, a walker will reduce the risk of falling down.

* If we cannot walk at all, we can still go nearly anywhere we want with an electric wheelchair. Some wheelchairs can even be raised up and down if we can't quite reach that upper shelf.

Some toilets are even equipped with automatic flushers, warm-water faucets for "personal cleansing," and air dryers—all to help people remain independent who would otherwise need assistance on the toilet.

Many of the items mentioned above are simply part of modern life, accessible to everyone and used by many. Even though you may get more exercise by taking the stairs, the elevator is generally available for everyone to enjoy. In addition, many types of specialized equipment are available to help people cope with disability or disease. For example, very elegant systems have been designed to allow people to live for decades with incontinence or even with a colostomy bag.

WE HAVE BETTER MEDICATION THAN EVER BEFORE

It is really very impressive to consider how many aspects of our lives can be improved by some kind of medication. If you have problems with high blood pressure you can reduce the risk of stroke or infarction with medication. The same goes for diabetes, depression, gout, arthritis, and heart disease. Many people with chronic conditions can now live quite comfortably if they have the right medication. Since chronic diseases are most frequently connected with the second half of life, this means medications often help people survive into old age.

WE HAVE MORE ORGANIZED HELP/ASSISTANCE THAN EVER BEFORE

Sometimes situations arise that we can't handle even with the right equipment, or maybe the right equipment doesn't exist yet. In these cases we may need the assistance of others. It may take a bit of their time to help us out, but often with some assistance we can move through a challenging situation and be independent again afterward.

Everyone needs help occasionally, not just older people. You yourself have probably asked for and received help while learning a new computer program, or using the escalator with children and shopping bags in tow, or getting your car out of a snowdrift. When we find ourselves in unusual situations, it is considered normal and desirable to ask for help to get ourselves back on track. We are not "burdening" others when we ask for a little assistance now and then; rather, we are offering them an opportunity to be of service. More than once you have probably stopped whatever you were doing to help a friend or even a stranger in need. Helping someone else may have even helped you feel good about yourself.

The kind of help or assistance we need in old age may be related to everyday life. Imagine that you suffer from arthritis and have a hard time putting on your socks. Of course, there is a grip-tool designed for just this situation, but your hands are too weak to use it. So for a few minutes every day you need assistance. For the rest of your day you are quite fine living on your own. In many communities, networks of organized help are available for older people, such as Meals on Wheels, senior citizen centers, organized volunteer services, and assisted-living facilities, to name a few.

WE CAN PROVIDE BETTER CARE THAN EVER BEFORE

The difference between assistance and care is that assistance covers only part of a procedure; the rest can be done independently. If a person is too weak or too sick to handle an entire procedure independently, he or she needs care. What, exactly, is long-term care? It is care designed to meet basic physical needs for activities of daily living (ADLs). ADLs may include everything from preparing meals to bathing to assistance using the toilet.

Imagine you have just woken up after having surgery. You want to go to the bathroom but your legs are too wobbly. You feel too weak to even sit up or wash yourself. You can't even think about getting dressed. On these days, you need care. If your postsurgical state of weakness is not expected to improve, you may need care for the rest of your life.

If something like this happens to your parents, it will be you who gets the phone call. The decision you make about how to care for them may impact you for several weeks or months. In fact, even if your parents' conditions are severely impaired, nowadays they could conceivably remain alive for quite a while, and this means your decision may impact you for years.

Improvements in Living Conditions

As discussed earlier, even if we suffer dramatically impaired health our potential lifespan has been greatly extended. Apart from better medical treatment, other basic living conditions have improved tremendously in the last century, making today's long-term care extremely successful at prolonging life. Today we can provide better environmental conditions, better hygiene conditions, and better nutritional conditions.

BETTER ENVIRONMENTAL CONDITIONS

Central heating and air conditioning now allow us to keep the external environment stable not only during the caring process but throughout the older patient's entire life. In quality, modern long-term-care facilities, the air conditioning systems are regularly maintained and kept sanitary to prevent the spread of disease that sometimes occurs when air ducts and filters are not regularly cleaned. The weakened elderly body no longer has to struggle with heat or cold. It is not exposed to extreme temperature changes, and the danger of getting a cold or secondary infection is reduced. The energy spent in controlling the room's climate directly results in life energy the older person can save by not having to fight temperature changes.

BETTER HYGIENE CONDITIONS

We now know that it is neither possible nor desirable to keep an elderly patient living under entirely aseptic conditions. But we do know how to prevent unnecessary infections. We know how to clean a room in a nursing home without bringing in bacteria from the neighbor's room simply by changing the towel. We know how to treat the bedridden patient's incontinence without causing skin infections and ulcers. We know how to reduce the likelihood of being exposed to harmful bacteria or viruses. In short, we know much more about how to provide a clean and healthful environment than we did just two or three decades ago.

BETTER NUTRITIONAL CONDITIONS

Some diseases require that the patient receive artificial nutrition, which normally means providing nutrition through a tube inserted directly through the abdomen into the stomach. Just a decade ago this procedure was quite rare; the surgery risk was considered higher than the likelihood of success. Instead, in a painful procedure the tube was inserted through the nose and throat directly into the gullet. Nowadays, with refined anesthesia and surgical methods, the risks stemming from inserting a feeding tube abdominally are rather low and inserting such a tube can mean several more months or years of life for the patient.

In addition, many forms of nutritionally balanced and complete liquid meals are available. Liquid foods can be sipped by those who are too weak to chew or who have chewing problems due to a stroke or Parkinson's disease. Thanks to liquid meals, many of the most severely ill elderly patients are consuming a more balanced diet than their fast-food-eating adult sons or daughters.

What Long-Term Care *Really* Looks Like

Current standards of living and recent advances in medical care have allowed us to come a long way from the "poor houses" of old. We have now come to think of long-term care as doing the best we can to meet a person's psychological and physical needs for as long as possible.

In the broadest sense of the word, "caring" means "taking over processes of self-preservation" for another person who is unable to do it for himself or herself. When we "care" for adults, it is usually due to sickness, weakness, or some mental disability associated with aging. But what does all of this caring look like? To see one example, let's revisit Gwen, the mother of Beth, the gardener, whom we met in the last chapter:

> Following her stroke, Gwen cannot move the entire right side
> of her body, including her head. That means she cannot fully
> move her mouth. Her ability to smile the grateful smile Beth

has imagined is not merely reduced but has been completely lost. Gwen can no longer use facial expressions to convey any emotions at all. The left side of the brain controls the right side of the body, and vice versa. Gwen's problem is on the left side of her brain, which is why the right side of her body is affected. Gwen has always been right-handed, so she is accustomed to handling important things with her right hand, which is now paralyzed.

Gwen's language center is also located on the damaged left side of her brain. This means she can no longer communicate through speech. She may even have lost the knowledge of the meanings of words. She may have to relearn language altogether. She may no longer understand simple questions such as, "Would you like some tea?" She looks at Beth as though Beth is speaking a foreign language. That's because to Gwen, Beth is speaking a foreign language.

That's not all. Gwen has problems swallowing food—even if it is mashed or in liquid form. She frequently coughs, spits up, and chokes. She cannot control her bladder or her sphincter. She suffers widespread muscular cramps that she cannot respond to or tell anyone about. Meanwhile, her mobile left side is caught in this sick body and feels like it has been strapped in for a long-distance flight for the remainder of its life.

Only thirty years ago, Gwen would have been condemned to staying in bed. She probably would have died within a few days due to her inability to eat. If she did manage to survive beyond that time she would quickly have developed bedsores and her feet would have become permanently crippled within a matter of weeks. Today, however, Gwen can be transferred from her bed to a wheelchair with the help of two trained people and some special equipment. Her wheelchair is adjusted to her exact proportions and protects her from falling or slipping over onto her weak side, where she cannot correct herself. So far she remains unable to handle her wheelchair. When she tries, she crashes into furniture or people. This occurs because her orientation was also affected by the stroke.

A special diaper system for adults helps Gwen stay as clean as possible. It keeps her from feeling wet and from developing skin rashes. The diapers have to be changed at least four times a day. More than once a day they may contain not just urine but also fecal matter. When this happens, it is necessary to wash Gwen's entire genital area and probably to change her clothes as well, since the diapers sometimes leak.

When she is in her wheelchair, Gwen sits on a special pillow that helps to distribute her body weight evenly so the risk of getting sores caused by permanent pressure is minimized. For the same reason, when she is in bed, Gwen has to be moved at least every two hours, even throughout the night.

Due to the dangers of choking on food or drink, someone in Gwen's condition may have a stomach tube inserted at the hospital. If this is the case, Gwen will have to be kept from moving in ways that could tear the incision. It will also become important for her caretaker to constantly monitor the consistency of the nutrition she will be given and the speed with which it will pass through the tube. This is true even for tea or water. Giving too much too fast or at the wrong consistency could cause Gwen to suffer a reflux reaction in her stomach. At some point, even if she is receiving nutrition through her feeding tube, Gwen will need to learn to swallow again. She will need to be retrained gradually, using small spoonfuls of liquid or mush.

Gwen should receive some kind of toilet training if her abilities are going to improve. For a while, after each meal, Gwen has to be transferred to the toilet with the help of two people. One of them has to stay with her while she is on the toilet to prevent her from sliding onto the floor. Her paralyzed right side will also have to be actively trained and passively massaged daily.

Since Gwen is taking (and needing) lots of naps during the day, she will be awake for long periods at night. She may lose her sense of time. Minutes will seem like eternity. Maybe she will start to scream if her caretaker leaves the room for more than just a moment. Or maybe she will simply feel lonely and uncomfortable.

There are many moments when Gwen seems to feel comfortable, even happy. During these times she looks very relaxed and attentive. Sometimes she even says a few unintelligible words. But if you ask her to repeat them, she will just stare at you, wondering what you are talking about.

Gwen may continue living for many months, even years. If you imagine what it will take to keep caring for Gwen, you will get some idea of the size of the job that's involved. Now you may have a better idea why long-term care has become a skilled profession.

If you really consider what is required to provide effective care for Gwen—the room, equipment, time, specialized knowledge, physical strength and vigor, endless patience, good humor, strong nerves, a strong stomach, and more—you will begin to see how Beth's instinctive decision to take her mother home with her is going to change her life in ways she has not yet begun to imagine. The next chapter examines in detail the implications of the decision to care for one's aging parents at home.

Chapter 4

The Home-Care Instinct

"When it became clear that my mother could no longer live alone, I brought her into our home to live with us," says Janet, age forty-seven. "I never considered any other place for her to live. I thought it would give her and me a chance to spend some quality time together, and I thought it would be good for the kids. I wanted them to learn respect for their elders. My plan was to demonstrate caring and compassion so they could see for themselves that families are supposed to take care of each other."

"Unfortunately, I think it has all backfired on me," Janet continues. "Mom complains about everything. Nothing we do is good enough. My husband, James, spends almost all his time at the office now just to be away from home. The kids don't hang around the house at all, and they never want to bring their friends over anymore. They say Grandma is disgusting, the way she coughs all the time and puts her dentures on the table during meals. I'm exhausted from trying to please everyone, and I feel like I made a big mistake. I love my mother, but if I had to do it all over again I think I'd find a different living arrangement for her."

The last chapter described many of the changes that have impacted the way we age and the way we care for our elders. It examined several of the reasons why it's not so easy to bring Mom or Dad home to our place to live out their remaining years. Most of these circumstances are only a few decades old and were completely unforeseen by everyone, save for a few academics who were ignored by the media. Thus, our society has not fully prepared for these changes, which is why discussions of Social Security and Medicare benefits headline many elections. Nor are we prepared for them as individuals. Most of us still operate under the social codes and beliefs we absorbed as children, neither of which are very good for dealing with the situations of today but both of which make us *feel* certain ways about the things we do.

Even when we know all the facts and figures, we don't necessarily feel any better about making the decision to place someone we love in a nursing home. Sure, the equipment there is better and they have trained staff, but we could just rent the equipment and hire some nurses' aides to come to our home—right? Nursing homes are for people who don't have anywhere else to go—aren't they? Isn't it *always* better to have your parent or loved one at home?

Home Care as a First Impulse

As caring human beings, our first inclination is often to bring our parent home to live with us, if at all possible. It is a protective impulse. Someone who took care of us now needs care, and we want to be there for him or her. We want to be near our parents and take care of them. We want to show our parents, ourselves, and maybe even our family and friends how much we care. Sometimes we feel a need to bring our loved one into our home because it is the "right" thing to do.

> "To bring Mom home" was Athena's immediate impulse after she got an emergency phone call at the office one Wednesday morning. It was her mother's doctor on the phone. He told Athena that her mother, Anna, had been found at home after a heart attack and had been brought to the hospital. Although the doctor expected Anna to survive, Anna had refused to accept a pacemaker. She also looked frail to him, as though she hadn't been eating well. He felt she would no longer be able to live alone.

As a businesswoman with a lot of responsibility, Athena was used to making quick decisions and taking action. She asked her assistant to book her a Friday-evening flight to her mother's city. Then she automatically began making plans for Anna to come live with her. Both Athena and her husband, Joe, agreed that it was unthinkable to place their parents in any kind of institution. In their social circles, that was something that simply wasn't done.

Before her trip, Athena had a carpenter widen the doorways to the bathroom and guest bedroom. She purchased a hospital bed and ordered an additional television set to be delivered over the weekend. She arranged for hired caregivers to attend to Anna during work days, and she tried to set aside a few hours in her busy schedule to spend with her mother during the next few months.

Athena was certain her mother would appreciate her efforts, and she was equally certain her mother would love the beautiful Italian designer sofas that Athena had purchased last month. Of course, there was no way Anna could bring her awful dog, Barky, along—but once Anna saw how wonderful Athena's home was, she would understand. Getting rid of the dog would be a small price for Anna to pay to come live with Athena and Joe.

Athena made a spontaneous decision to bring her mother home. Once the decision was made, she never really gave it a second thought. She was too busy. Besides, she didn't believe there was any viable alternative. Still, it might have been worthwhile for Athena to explore whether or not she was truly ready to have her mother live with her, and to investigate what exactly "bringing Mother home" might mean.

What Does "Home" Mean?

To Athena, bringing her mother home meant little more than finding a place for Anna in her already overbooked schedule. But what does it mean to be "at home"? Are you at home in the same way at your son's or daughter's house as you are at your own house? Like you, your elderly loved ones have their own place in the world, and it may be difficult for them to think of the place where you live as their "home."

We live in a very mobile society. Our friends and family members may change addresses frequently. Many of us have lived in several different places. Sometimes we live in places where we don't feel at home at all, whether it is with our parents and siblings or maybe even in our hometown. It's very possible that when Athena and her mother, Anna, think of home, they think of two entirely different things. For Athena, being at home means being surrounded by nice material belongings, such as her Italian sofas. It also means being with her husband, Joe, and being respected by those in her social environment.

> When Athena finally walked into her mother's hospital room, she was shocked at the sight of her mother lying in bed with tubes and wires connected to her body. Anna looked a lot more frail than Athena had imagined she would, but she kissed her mother quickly and reassured her that there was nothing to worry about. She proudly told Anna that all the preparations had been made for her to come live with them. She spoke with confidence. Athena was 100-percent sure that Anna would be relieved and would feel pride in and gratitude toward her hardworking, successful daughter.
>
> Anna listened until Athena finished talking. Then she smiled and said, "No, thank you." She preferred to go to a local assisted-living facility instead! Anna explained that she had applied for a room in the facility some months ago, and by good fortune one had just come available last week. Several of her friends were already residents there, and Anna was looking forward to the move.
>
> Athena was still in shock when Anna asked for "just one small favor." "Yes, of course. Anything!" Athena replied. So Anna asked Athena to take her dog, Barky, back home to live with Athena and Joe. Anna couldn't take Barky to her new place, and she couldn't bear to think of her precious pet going to live with a stranger.

Within a day of arriving at the hospital, Athena was on a plane headed back home. Barky was in a crate in the hold of the plane, and Athena was fuming. No mother of hers belonged in a home!

For Anna, to be "at home" had a lot to do with the material environment, but it was not her house that Anna considered home; rather, it was her hometown. She wanted to be near her friends and the places that had mattered to her over the years. Both Anna and Athena considered the social environment when defining "home" for themselves, but what was home to Athena was not home to Anna.

If your parent is conscious and mentally alert, chances are he or she has some pretty strong ideas about what he or she considers home. It may be prudent to ask so you can find out what these ideas are.

Exercise: What Does "Home" Mean?

We encourage you to take a few moments on your own to do the following exercise. Answer the questions as completely as you can. Avoid censoring your ideas; just write them down quickly and without judgment. Answer with specifics whenever you can. For example, if your hometown is one of the important elements that mean "home" to you, don't just write "my hometown." Write the name of the town, for example, "Redford, Michigan." If being near friends is an important factor, write down the names of the friends you want to be near, for example, "Tom Wilson." If you don't want to write in this book, use a separate sheet of paper or a journal.

If you need help coming up with answers to the questions, consider these six categories:

* Physical places (specific dwellings, buildings, parks, campuses)

* Possessions and pets (your favorite chair, animal, stamp collection)

* Certain people (specific friends, family members, teachers, colleagues, doctors, therapists)

* Special experiences, traditions, and memories (childhood memories, first date, first kiss, holiday activities)

* Specific activities (work/job, volunteer work, hobbies, exercise routines, sports)

* Communities (social clubs, teams, religious or spiritual congregations, neighborhood gathering spots)

1. When I think of "home," I think of the following things (list at least six things—more if you can):

_____

_____

_____

_____

_____

_____

2. When my parent thinks of "home," he or she *probably* thinks of the following things (if possible, consider asking your parent to answer this question. If your parent can no longer respond for herself or himself, discuss it with his or her friends or your siblings to gain a broader perspective):

_____

_____

_____

_____

_____

_____

Look at your answers to the two questions above. Put an X beside any differences in the two lists, such as different hometowns or different ideas of what matters. It is important for you to be aware of these differences when you make a long-term-care decision on behalf of your parent.

3. What kinds of things might your parent expect or require from his or her home? (If you get stuck here, think of the things that *you* might want if you were in your parent's condition, such as physical comfort, clean surroundings, special medical equipment, etc.):

_____

_____

_____

_____

_____

_____

_____

4. Take a look at the list you made in answering question 3 and ask yourself the following two questions:

a. Can I honestly provide all of the things that my parent will need or expect in a home if I bring my parent home to live with me?

Yes   No

b. Do I genuinely want to provide all these things?

Yes   No

Think about your answers to questions 4a and 4b to make sure you are being fully honest with yourself. No one else needs to see this worksheet, so be true to your real feelings. Unless both answers are a solid yes, you may want to consider alternatives to caring for your parent in your own home. We will discuss some of those alternatives in Chapter 6. If you replied yes to 4a but no to 4b, and if you have any uncomfortable feelings about that discrepancy, keep reading. We will discuss these uncomfortable emotions in the next chapter, "Your Feelings Matter More than You May Think."

If you are still leaning toward bringing your mother or father home to live with you, be sure to read the next chapter to get very clear about your reasons why. You'll want to rule out some of the more harmful reasons for wanting to do so (e.g., a belief that you have no choice, instinctive dependency, wanting social approval, unconsciously wanting revenge). For now, there are a few more related issues to consider:

* Your loved one's condition
* Your energy level
* The need for community
* The economics of home care
* Finding balance between serving others and serving yourself

Most of the rest of this chapter is devoted to examining these issues. The chapter ends with a detailed exercise, "Are You Ready for Home Care?" that will help you take all these factors into account when considering your options.

Your Loved One's Condition

Perhaps you are considering bringing your mother home to live with you after the recent death of your father. Aside from being in mourning and feeling sad, your mother is in good physical and emotional health. Your relationship with her has been easy, pleasant, and relaxed for many years, as has her relationship with your spouse and children. You have enough room in your home for everyone to cohabit comfortably and with adequate privacy, and your intention is a loving one, based solely on wanting to ease her loneliness now that she is a widow. You have plenty of time to spend with her and sufficient resources to share. She has been consulted and is eager, or at least willing, to move in with you, and you are looking forward to having her there.

If what you have just read applies to you, that's terrific. You are in an excellent situation to enjoy a successful home-care relationship with your mother. But what if your situation varies somewhat from the ideal, as many do? If your relationship with your mother has been troubled, it is not likely to improve under the stress of her making a major move and your family's having to adjust to having a new resident in the house.

In the next chapter we'll discuss feelings about your parents that you may have been repressing, such as resentment or anger or even a desire for revenge. Feelings like these can lead to hostile and even abusive relationships, or to illness in either person. We have also mentioned how important it is that everyone living in your home be a partner in the home-care decision to the greatest extent possible, and we have discussed the pitfalls of trying to make a decision on behalf of your parent without consulting him or her. Now we need to take a closer look at your mother's or father's physical and mental condition. If your situation is similar to that of Beth, whose mother, Gwen, just suffered a stroke, your parent is going to need around-the-clock skilled nursing care. Beth will need to determine what she really wants to do about Gwen's care, and in doing so she will need to look at the reality of Gwen's physical condition.

Consider your loved one's condition very carefully before making the decision to bring him or her into your home. Equally important, think about how his or her condition is likely to change in the future. If your parent needs special equipment, training, or medical care to keep him or her safe and comfortable, you have a lot of evaluating to do.

Your Energy Level

We each have a certain amount of life energy. For the purposes of this example, think of your personal energy as being stored in an "energy bank." You "spend" the energy out of your "bank" to accomplish three things:

1. To stay alive

2. To develop and improve yourself

3. To give some energy to others

Consider the energy that is required to care for an older person. Who will provide that energy? In times past, the typical family had several children who could each contribute to caring for a parent or grandparent. These days, families tend to be much smaller. If only one child is responsible for the care of a parent, that child must provide all the energy involved in the care while still maintaining his or her own livelihood, health, and well-being.

In the right circumstances, caring for other people can replenish your energy. You may feel uplifted and energized by the experience; you may learn and grow from it. Most people, for example, find parenting their children to be rewarding in this way. Caring for a parent can be a character-building experience as well. You may discover things about yourself and your abilities that you never realized. On the other hand, caring for someone else can take energy away from your own needs. New parents who don't get to sleep through the night for several months tend to be less energetic than they were before the baby came along. When you are caring for a parent it is important to avoid putting yourself in a position where you withdraw too much of the energy from your life's "bank" that you need for your own survival. You have to take care of yourself and your own health, too.

Let's look at the energy required to provide home care for an aging parent from the perspective of simple mathematics and logic. An extremely sick person, like Beth's mother, Gwen, can need up to 24 hours of care and attention per day, which equals 168 hours per week. Any professional caregivers who are hired will work a normal 40-hour week. So this means 4.2 full-time caregivers will be needed in order to provide around-the-clock care. But the caregivers will need time off for vacations, holidays, occasional sick days, and professional training. They will also require some over-lapping time at the beginning and end of each shift to communicate with each other about the patient's needs. It follows, then, that one very sick person may need the time and attention of up to 5 or 6 different full-time caregivers on an ongoing basis. This may sound like an exaggeration. Trust us—it's not. Xenia's years of staffing nursing homes and Lynn's experience helping to line up in-home caregivers for her mother-in-law, who has Alzheimer's, back up these figures.

In the preindustrial-age family, the home-care "staff" consisted of older children, unmarried sisters, and possibly some servants, and their help was needed for a relatively short span of years. If your parent is seriously ill, and you have five or six family members who are willing to devote their energy full-time to caring for him or her, possibly for many years, you can make home care work. If there are fewer than five of you caring for your ailing parent, you could be endangering your own health. You may never know the full extent of the consequences to your body of taking on such a serious responsibility.

The Need for Community

The amount of social contact each person needs varies from person to person, but almost everyone requires a certain amount of interpersonal interaction. Participation in a community gives us a sense of belonging, a sense of importance, and a sense of meaning. But not all communities are created equal. As we saw with Athena's mother, Anna, a network of friends is as important to many elderly people as it is to younger ones, and even the most adoring of grandchildren can't replace a long-term friendship with a peer. Over time, home care often enriches the relationship between parent and child. Still, no one person can fulfill all the social needs of another. The larger the potential community, the more choices one has about whom to spend time with. If you are considering home care for your loved one, be sure to take into account his or her need for social contact. Too many home-care situations turn into something akin to solitary confinement for the elderly person.

Concerns about the need for community are not restricted only to the patient. Home caregivers may find their own social interactions drastically altered. If you are fond of going out with friends, you may find this activity (and these friendships) severely impacted by taking in your elderly parent. On the other hand, if you do not spend much time in social pursuits, providing home care for a parent can open up new avenues of contact with others through support groups designed specifically for caregivers (see the Resources section, located in the back of this book, for information on such groups). And be sure to fully consider the pros and cons of your social habits and needs before making any decisions about long-term in-home care.

The Economics of Home Care

Sometimes people consider home care because they believe it will be less expensive than institutionalized care. Depending on certain factors, including your loved one's condition, this may or may not be true. We have already seen that quality home care can require up to five additional people to look after an ailing patient. If you don't have the agreement of specific family members that they will be involved in providing care, those extra people will have to be hired. If your parent needs specialized health care, you will need to hire skilled workers, who will charge more than if your parent is self-sufficient. And then there are the normal costs of everyday living associated with having another person in the household, such as meals (perhaps involving special nutritional considerations), clothing, and increased utility bills.

We have prepared the following worksheet to help you determine if providing home care makes financial sense for you. Fill in only the fields that apply to your situation. For example, if bringing your parent home to live with you will not cost anything in terms of accommodations, leave that row blank. On the other hand, if you will have to modify your home to allow for wheelchair access, or otherwise upgrade or refurnish the room your parent will occupy, estimate the total cost of the modifications and write that number under "One-time costs" in the "Accommodations" row. If you are moving into your parent's home to care for him or her and if this will involve monthly rent or mortgage costs, list these under "Cost per month."

In each of the rows for hired aides, you will have to determine both the number of hours you are likely to need help and the cost of help in your geographical area. If the help needed is purely physical, it will be less costly than if nursing or other medical help is necessary. We have included a row labeled "Senior day care." For a discussion of this topic, see the section that appears later in this chapter.

Some costs for medical equipment are one-time costs, such as wheelchair, walker, lifter, or hospital bed. Others are ongoing, such as diapers, blood-testing strips for diabetics, and gauze. Use the appropriate row to estimate both types of costs for your situation.

The columns labeled "Covered by?" allow you to indicate who is paying for a particular cost. Some costs may be covered by health, disability, or long-term-care insurance; some by your parent's own assets such as pension, investment, or Social Security income; some by Medicare; some by a relative; and some by you. There are multiple columns to accommodate expenses that will be partially covered by different sources. For example, perhaps your mother's health insurance covers her prescriptions but she has a deductible or co-pay. In each case, be sure to record where the money is coming from and how much it is likely to be.

We advise you to guess high in your estimates; in general things will cost more rather than less than you think. In creating this worksheet we have not thought of every possible scenario. We intended it to be a starting point from which you can gain some idea of the likely costs involved in your particular home-care situation. (This chart and others in this book may be reproduced for personal use. They can be enlarged to 130% and will fit on a normal letter-size sheet.)

Cost of Care Worksheet

TYPE OF COST	Hours per day	Hours per week	Hours per month	Cost per month	One-time costs	Covered by?	Covered by?	Covered by?
Accommodations								
Meals								
Housekeeping								
Morning aide								
Noon aide								
Evening aide								
Medical treatment								
Bathing aide								
Night aide								
Senior day care								
Medical equipment (one-time expenses)								
Medical equipment (ongoing)								
Totals								

Serving Others Versus Serving Yourself: Finding the Balance

Bringing up our children and taking care of our parents are both very basic biological and social survival strategies. But most cultural, social, philosophical, and religious belief systems tell us that there is more to life than just fulfilling these two tasks. Most widespread systems of thought have at their root a belief that each person's gifts and talents are unique. If this is true, any person who does not fully develop or use his or her talents is depriving the world.

You may find yourself in a situation similar to Beth's, whose mother, Gwen, had a stroke just as Beth was dreaming of finally following her passion for gardening. Perhaps you have already devoted a portion of your life to caring for your family, deferring the development of some of your own talents until recently—and now your spouse or elderly parent needs care. It can be challenging to determine where to draw the line between taking care of yourself and taking care of others.

If you believe that your talents were given to you for a reason, then it follows that you are responsible for developing and sharing them with the world as well as you possibly can. If you have your own dreams, passions, or career, it is important to consider how in-home elder-care will impact those facets of your life. If your gifts and interests naturally involve caring for others, if you are drawn to health- and/or counseling-related subjects, and if you have intentionally made your family the centerpiece of your life until now, you may find yourself well suited to caring for your parent at home. You are quite likely to find the experience satisfying, gratifying, and even energizing. If you have these natural inclinations and are presently working in a career that does not maximize them, you may even find it more fulfilling to leave your job and care for your parent at home.

But what if your personal gifts run along very different lines? Perhaps you are given to more artistic or commercial pursuits. Maybe you are passionate about sailing or accounting or making music. If so, then consider very carefully whether in-home elder-care will allow you to make the most of your innate abilities or whether it will impede them. As we have pointed out, elder-care these days is likely to last for several years. How will you feel if you need to defer your dreams entirely in order to become an in-home, skilled nursing professional?

It is not selfish to want to maximize the gifts you were born with and the opportunities you have to use them. It is okay to admit if you are not the right type of personality to happily care for your parent at home. Not only is it okay; it is essential to your well-being and the well-being of your family, including your aging loved one. Too many elders are subject to abusive comments or worse from resentful children (or their children's spouses) who are caring for "Mom" or "Dad" at home when they would rather be elsewhere following their own dreams.

When our parents need our help, we don't have to see it as an either/or situation. We don't have to give up our dreams to care for the ones we love. Nor do we have to shirk our responsibility in caring for them to live our dreams. In situations like Beth's, alternatives are available. She could find one that will both allow her mother to receive trained, professional help for the twenty-four hours each day she needs it *and* allow Beth to pursue her dreams. Both parties can get what they need, and both sets of needs can be pursued with a motivation of love.

A Note about Senior Day Care

Senior day care is a rapidly growing industry that caters to those who are caring for their elderly parents at home. As the name implies, senior-day-care centers are designed to allow home caregivers to leave their parents at the center during the day. Services vary from center to center, but most provide activities, companionship, and midday meals and/or snacks. The older person gets to experience an expanded sense of community, and the home caregiver can continue working at an outside job or caring for young children who need full attention during the day. If you are considering home care, a quality senior-day-care center will allow you to pursue your daytime activities while knowing that your parent is being well looked after and also that he or she has an opportunity for enjoying friendships with other people during the day.

While senior day care can be an excellent addition to the home-care routine, it is not a complete solution for caring for your elderly parent. For one thing, it isn't yet available everywhere. In addition, many senior-day-care centers target a specific ethnic or cultural community; they may even use the native language of the group during activities and interaction. This may or may not be compatible with your own loved one's needs. Furthermore, depending on where you live, senior day care can be prohibitively expensive.

If senior day care that can accommodate your needs and those of your parent is available in your area, be aware that you will still need extra support at home. To get your parent ready for day care in the morning, you will need to see that he or she is toileted, washed, and dressed before leaving the house, which may mean adding a considerable amount of time to your morning routine before you leave for work. After work, when you pick up your parent, you will still be responsible for feeding, toileting, and preparing him or her for bed—at which point you are working the night shift. If you rely on senior day care you may have to miss a day or more of work occasionally if your parent is sick or is unable or unwilling to attend the center. If your job will be threatened by such a possibility, be sure to have backup care lined up for such situations. Senior day care will allow you to continue working, but, depending on your parent's condition, you may still need additional home-care workers to assist you during your nonworking hours.

Exercise: Are You Ready for Home Care?

Answer the questions below to determine whether your "home-care instinct" is more than just an instinct. Does it have a realistic chance of working for you and your family? Using the number 1 to represent statements that are "absolutely false" and the number 7 to represent those that are "absolutely true," circle the number that best describes your level of agreement or disagreement with each statement below.

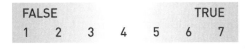

My Body

It is one thing to see your loved one at Thanksgiving once a year and quite another to be awakened three times a night by an elderly parent who needs to be comforted or needs help going to the toilet.

1. I am in excellent health.	1 2 3 4 5 6 7
2. I have a lot of extra energy.	1 2 3 4 5 6 7
3. I have no back or shoulder problems.	1 2 3 4 5 6 7
4. I am not overweight.	1 2 3 4 5 6 7
5. I can easily bend over and squat.	1 2 3 4 5 6 7
6. I can work while resting on my knees.	1 2 3 4 5 6 7
7. I can handle having my sleep interrupted one or more times per night.	1 2 3 4 5 6 7
8. I have realistic ways to restore and renew my energy.	1 2 3 4 5 6 7
9. Someone will be there for my parent when I go to exercise or have a personal trainer come to my home.	1 2 3 4 5 6 7
10. Someone will be there for my parent so I can take breaks during the hours when I am caring for him or her.	1 2 3 4 5 6 7
11. I will have enough time to handle shopping and meal preparation.	1 2 3 4 5 6 7

My Heart and Soul

12. I can find somebody to take care of my loved one while I take an annual vacation.	1 2 3 4 5 6 7

13. There are no unresolved conflicts   1 2 3 4 5 6 7
between my parent and me.

14. I felt loved and appreciated as a child.   1 2 3 4 5 6 7

15. I handle frustration well.   1 2 3 4 5 6 7

16. I am ready to look clearly at the rela-   1 2 3 4 5 6 7
tionship I've had with my parent.

17. I am quite sure there are no old   1 2 3 4 5 6 7
conflicts hidden behind a friendly
façade between my loved one and me.

18. I can live without hearing a "thank   1 2 3 4 5 6 7
you" when I help someone.

19. I know where to find spiritual support,   1 2 3 4 5 6 7
good ideas, and understanding
people to talk to when I need a listening ear.

20. I know where to find a caregiver's   1 2 3 4 5 6 7
support group.

21. I am aware that the amount of energy   1 2 3 4 5 6 7
I will spend will probably never corre-
late to the appreciation I will get from
others.

My Family Support

At this stage of your life you are probably not just sitting around doing nothing. Your days are filled with activity. With a new caregiving task, some of the things you do now will have to be taken over by other family members.

22. I am not involved in supporting my   1 2 3 4 5 6 7
spouse's career by attending func-
tions or organizing events.

23. Over 50 percent of my time is free for   1 2 3 4 5 6 7
leisure activities.

24. My family members know what will   1 2 3 4 5 6 7
be expected of each of them—and
they all agree.

25. My spouse can live with my interrupt-   1 2 3 4 5 6 7
    ing his or her sleep one or more
    times each night.

My Knowledge

26. I am willing and able to learn about   1 2 3 4 5 6 7
    diseases and medication.

27. I like reading about medical issues.   1 2 3 4 5 6 7

28. I enjoy writing reports and detailed   1 2 3 4 5 6 7
    information for caregivers.

29. I am good at learning how to handle   1 2 3 4 5 6 7
    machines and technical equipment.

30. I have a good short-term memory.   1 2 3 4 5 6 7

My Home

Some elderly people, like Amy's mother, Ruth, develop nighttime dementia such as sundowner's syndrome. They may be quite normal during the day, but confused and disoriented at night. Occasionally, patients with dementia may soil themselves and play with their feces at night, dirtying walls and furniture.

31. I can easily move a wheelchair   1 2 3 4 5 6 7
    through the rooms of my house.

32. The floors can be easily cleaned after   1 2 3 4 5 6 7
    being contaminated by feces or urine.

33. The bathroom is on the same floor as   1 2 3 4 5 6 7
    my parent's room.

34. There are no steps or stairs that my   1 2 3 4 5 6 7
    parent will have to negotiate.

35. I can reach my parent's bed from both   1 2 3 4 5 6 7
    sides if necessary.

36. My parent's room has air conditioning   1 2 3 4 5 6 7
    and central heating.

37. The room is not furnished with easily   1 2 3 4 5 6 7
    damaged or expensive items.

My Equipment ———————————————

38. The room, the house, and the street   1 2 3 4 5 6 7
are accessible by wheelchair.

39. There is enough space for a lifter.   1 2 3 4 5 6 7

40. I know where to get a hospital bed.   1 2 3 4 5 6 7

41. Someone will be there to help lift and   1 2 3 4 5 6 7
transfer my parent from bed to
wheelchair, from wheelchair to
recliner.

My Social Environment ———————————

42. I am open to discussing even contro-   1 2 3 4 5 6 7
versial topics with my doctor.

43. I don't worry about what my neigh-   1 2 3 4 5 6 7
bors think of me.

44. My neighbors will support me even if   1 2 3 4 5 6 7
my parent is screaming at night (as
some elderly people do). They won't
worry about its effect on their real
estate values.

45. My neighbors will support me when I   1 2 3 4 5 6 7
need extra help.

46. My neighborhood is good for a walk   1 2 3 4 5 6 7
or a ride in a wheelchair.

Now total your points: _____

Less than 135: We strongly urge you not to consider home care in your present situation. It would not be in the best interest of you or your parent to bring him or her into your home. Instead, save your energy and develop a partnership with a good nursing home.

Between 135 and 225: Home care may or may not work for you. Find out about the positive aspects of nursing homes before you decide. If you opt for a home-care situation, be sure to organize a reliable support system of family members and professional caregivers.

More than 225: It's up to you! You can make the home-care decision or look for a good nursing home. It will still be worthwhile for you to at least explore all your options by reading the rest of this book.

WARNING—If you answer "no" to *any* of the five questions that follow, we strongly advise you not to consider a home-caring situation:

Note: You may feel as though many of the conditions listed below do not apply to your parent. Maybe your mother is not in a wheelchair or is not incontinent. Each person must evaluate his or her own parent's condition—*as well as the parent's likely future condition*—for him- or herself. We include this list because it shows the types of situations nursing home staff deal with every day with many of their residents.

1. Does it bother you to see feces or urine? To touch it? To smell it?

2. Does it bother you to see and smell expectorated (spit-up) material?

3. Can you listen to a person screaming or moaning for hours?

4. Do you suffer from any kind of depression, or have you in the past?

5. Did you feel neglected or were you abused by your parent?

CONSIDER YOUR CAREER

Will you have to give up your job to become a caregiver? If so, what sorts of benefits will you lose? Health insurance? Paid vacation? Paid sick days? Retirement savings potential?

If you are considering home care to save money, what would you earn if you kept your job instead of quitting it to provide home care? Or, if you're not currently working but would enjoy going back to work, what would you earn if you took a job instead of providing home care? Remember to consider the value of benefits such as Social Security contributions and pension plans, if they are applicable.

If after answering all these questions you still feel unsure about whether home care is right for you, it is important not to take action just yet. We suggest talking to a licensed professional counselor, social worker, clergy member, or therapist before making your decision. As a starting point for your discussions you may want to share your responses to these exercises with him or her.

Maybe We'll Just Give It a Try...

If you're not absolutely certain that home care is for you, keep exploring other options. It is difficult for an elderly person to move from one environment to another. Your mother or father will have to make a major adjustment. It will mean changes in his or her schedule, habits, routines, social contacts, and personal comforts. No matter where your parent moves, the move will be stressful and take energy. If you move your parent into your home on a "trial" basis and it doesn't work out, that means he or she will have to move again. Making two major moves and two major adjustments during his or her later years may very well exhaust your parent. Also, any chronic health condition your parent lives with may be exacerbated by the stress of a double move.

Your parent's—and your own—feelings also need to be considered. If you bring your parent home with you and it doesn't work out, he or she may feel even more betrayed, abandoned, or hurt than if he or she had gone right to a nursing home in the first place. You both may experience feelings of failure or shame, and as a result your relationship may suffer long-term damage.

In the next chapter you'll learn in depth why it is so important to be sensitive to people's feelings during the process of making the nursing home decision—your feelings, your parent's feelings, and your siblings' feelings. You'll explore different emotions that are commonly associated with putting a parent into a nursing home; you'll learn why you have these emotions and what you should do with them. You may discover some surprising things about yourself.

Chapter 5

Your Feelings Matter More than You May Think

*I can keep my feelings to myself. I can push them to the
side. But you have to realize, I can't make them go away.*

— *Terri Foster*

You may be surprised to find a chapter on feelings in this book,
when all you want is to figure out what to do about your aging
loved one. But after a lifetime of negative conditioning about nursing homes, you are probably experiencing many confusing emotions in response to the decision to place a parent in long-term
care. In this chapter we discuss the most common feelings that
arise during this challenging period of life. We help you define
what you are feeling, and we give you some sense of how your emotions may influence your behavior. Every person is unique, and we
all respond to situations differently. Read this chapter and do the
exercise to help you make sense of the particular mix of emotions
you're experiencing. You'll also learn something about what your
parent and perhaps even your other family members are going
through. When you make decisions with a clear sense of how you
and others feel, you have a much better chance of success. You're
able to see the little details concerning a nursing home in the most

appropriate light and to calmly make changes when the situation calls for it. You're better able to help your parent, other family members and residents, and yourself.

This chapter will help you put your emotions into words by offering suggestions for how to express them in a healthy and beneficial way when they become troublesome. Perhaps most important it will give you confidence. Confidence that what you are doing is the right thing. Confidence that your loved one will be well cared for. Confidence that your family's interactions near the end of your parent's life can be loving and fulfilling, perhaps for the first time in years. Take the time to work through the material in this chapter carefully. Doing so may be the best investment in time you make during this entire process—and it will pay off for years to come in the added benefit of enhanced emotional health.

Your Feelings Determine Your Experience

There are two major points of view to consider in creating a rewarding nursing home experience:

* For your loved one, the nursing home resident, the desired experience is living well *in* a nursing home.

* For you, the family member living outside, it is living well *with* a nursing home.

Although nursing homes are places to live and be happy *in*, they are usually sold to family members as places they can be happy *with*. General talk about the quality of nursing homes tends to focus on a lot of little details that can be seen, measured, and rated. These can be published in reports or presented in full-color, glossy brochures, but they are not necessarily the most important elements of a satisfying nursing home experience. How well you live with a nursing home will primarily be a question of two powerful, unseen factors. First, far more important than how many choices are offered to the residents at mealtime is how well you are able to cope with all the different emotions you have surrounding the idea of "Nursing Home." You'll also need to be adept at dealing with the complex feelings that are a part of your relationship with your parent. We consider your feelings, or the emotional part of your inner world, to be the most important thing you have to cope with when it comes to living well with a nursing home. Your emotions will function as the basis of all your other perceptions about the nursing home experience.

When people's feelings about any aspect concerning a certain subject are negative, they tend to regard everything about that subject as negative. Even a single event may be enough to cement their perceptions. If you have ill feelings about nursing homes in general, it will be very difficult for you to have a satisfactory experience with even the best of nursing homes. Your mother or father may be comfortable, well cared for, and happy there, but if you have a bad taste for nursing homes in general, you will always be looking for that little bit of dust on the highest shelf. When you find it, and you will, you'll use it as evidence that you were right all along about nursing homes being awful places, and you'll feel terrible about sending your mother or father to live in one. By contrast, if you feel neutral or good about nursing homes in general, then the occasional misunderstanding or minor problem will be easy for you to overlook or deal with calmly.

The second unseen factor that will influence your nursing home experience is what we call the *atmosphere* of a nursing home. Atmo-

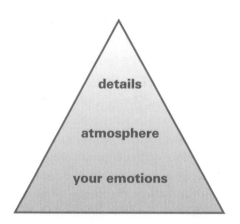

Figure 1. The most important factors to recognize when seeking a satisfying nursing home experience

sphere is what you intuitively respond to when you walk in and look around. You get a feeling for how the staff interacts with each other and with the residents. You also get a sense of the atmosphere when you watch most of the residents (and not just one small, active group) engaged in a variety of simple activities according to their abilities.

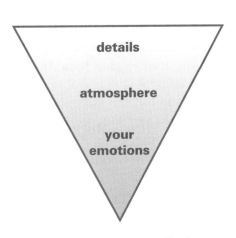

Figure 2. A problematic way of looking at factors relating to nursing homes

We do agree that the observable "details," such as the facility's equipment, are important. But from our point of view it works as illustrated in Figure 1.

Unfortunately, too many people operate under precisely the opposite assumption. Their triangle is inverted (see Figure 2). The details of the facility, such as attractive landscaping, take a place of paramount importance, and the emotional part of the situation is all too often overlooked.

This triangle will eventually crash down. It offers no stable basis for developing a good long-term relationship with either your parent or a nursing home. It only ensures that perception problems will persist between the important but much maligned institution known as a nursing home and the general public. Furthermore, if you are focused mainly on the details of your mother's or father's nursing home and are overlooking your feelings about the situation, your own state of affairs is in danger of falling apart in one way or another.

We think it's a really good idea—in fact, as we said earlier it may be the most important thing you can do—for all family members involved in the nursing home decision to become aware both of their emotions and attitudes toward each other and of their feelings toward nursing homes and aging in general. Only then do we suggest taking the next steps toward making the nursing home decision.

The Nature of Emotions

Decisions about how to care for our aging parents are inevitably fraught with emotion. Whether we have visited our parents every day or haven't spoken to them in years, at least on the emotional level we have interacted with them all our lives. Sometimes the complex feelings we have may seem to contradict one another. For example, you may feel a sense of relief mixed with guilt when placing a loved one in a nursing home.

Unfortunately, most of us were not taught the skills of emotional literacy in school. Many otherwise very intelligent people regard their emotions as rather foreign and mysterious, if they think about them at all. Feelings can be difficult to understand. It may sometimes seem as though they are controlling you, as if they are responsible for your behavior. At times you may have no idea what to call the emotion you are feeling or why you are feeling it. You may have trouble knowing what to do with your emotions.

The good news is you are *not* your feelings. You are a person who has feelings. You may be unable to consciously choose how you feel, but you *can* choose what to do with your feelings. The choices you make about how you express your emotions will make a world of difference in how you and your parent experience the long-term-care decision.

We humans often feel the need to share our feelings with others. We always have a choice of how we do this. If we choose to express our feelings in a sincere, honest, and respectful way, we are likely to help heal ourselves and our relationships. If we choose instead to express our feelings by playing the victim or martyr, or by pointing fingers and finding fault, or by making others feel they are wrong and putting them on the defensive, we are likely to make the situation more difficult for everyone involved.

People respond to situations differently. In one family we knew, two adult sisters took turns visiting their mother in a nursing home. When Keesha visited her mother one day, she noticed that her mother's sock drawer seemed to be missing some socks. Keesha got upset and complained loudly and bitterly to the nurse's aide. She said accusatory and insulting things. Her visit to her mother was tarnished with ill feelings, and the sock drawer was unaffected by her tirade.

The next day, when Kanya visited, she also noticed that her mother's sock drawer seemed to be missing a few pairs. Kanya realized that she herself sometimes lost socks in the wash at home, and she made a mental note to pick up a few new pairs of socks for her mother before her next visit. Kanya's visit to see her mother was pleasant and uplifting for both of them, and in a couple of days the sock drawer was full again.

The situation was the same, but Keesha and Kanya responded to it differently. Keesha felt an uncomfortable emotion, possibly some guilt or sadness over having placed her mother in a nursing home. To avoid feeling any pain triggered by her guilt or sadness, she refused to acknowledge her feelings, instead transforming them into upset and blame aimed at the poor nurse's aide. Kanya, who had a clearer sense of her own feelings, was able remain detached about the missing socks. She realized that no one was really to blame. Sometimes socks just disappear in the wash. She solved the problem on another level: by buying new socks for her mother. Each woman made a choice about how to respond to the same situation. Keesha's choice may have been unconscious on her part, and she may not have owned it as a choice, but it was a choice nonetheless. She didn't have to act the way she did. She chose to behave that way.

If a situation triggers feelings of anger or frustration in you, make careful and respectful decisions about how you choose to express these emotions. You're far more likely to get what you want with a controlled response than if you lose your temper or blame another person for your state of mind. As mentioned previously, in the next section we'll talk more about specific strategies for expressing various emotions. For now, just know that you have a choice about how to do so. Know also that your choice will have an effect on your experience and, therefore, on your level of satisfaction with any interaction.

What You May Be Feeling about the Nursing Home Decision

In this section we'll explore some of the most common feelings that arise when people learn they must begin making certain care decisions for their parent or parents. You may experience one or even all of these emotions at some point in your decision-making process. We hope the information provided here will give you some tools for recognizing your feelings and deciding what to do with them.

CONFUSION

When you feel the first impulse to take care of your parent in whatever way it occurs to you to do so, you may momentarily forget that you also have other priorities. When priorities seem to conflict with one another, the result is confusion. Perhaps your first instinct is to bring your parent into your home, but then you remember that your spouse or children may have some thoughts about the matter. What do you do in the face of conflicting desires? Where do your deepest loyalties lie? That's the situation Bert, the doctor from Chapter 2, ran into when he first had the idea to bring his estranged, alcoholic father, Albert, into his home. Bert's decision to bring Albert home may have had something to do with his wanting to "fix" things between himself and his father, but what about the relationship between Bert and his wife, Susan?

> When Bert told Susan that he wanted Albert to come live with them, her response was very clear: "There is absolutely no way!" She gave Bert an ultimatum: If he brought Albert into

their home, she would move out immediately. She had already been feeling neglected by Bert, and now she was afraid he would pay more attention to Albert than to her. Bert knew he had a decision to make. But what to decide? On the one hand, he had years of issues to work out with Albert, and this could be his last chance. On the other, he very much wanted his marriage to survive, and he now realized it needed some work too.

After sleeping on it that night (probably on the sofa), Bert decided to find another home for Albert. He also resolved to work on improving the communication in his marriage. By making this decision, and without even knowing it, Bert took the first step toward healing the wounds he had been carrying since childhood, wounds he had always blamed Albert for inflicting upon him.

Bert says, "I'm glad things worked out this way. I never realized Susan was so unhappy in our marriage. Now that I know, I can try to do something about it." As for Albert, he manages to walk the two blocks from his new retirement home to the local bar nearly every day. The bar is where he feels most at home.

You may be dealing with a similar situation. Perhaps you think you want to bring your parent home so you can care for him or her in your own environment. But unless you live alone, the decision is not solely yours. Your spouse and, if applicable, your children must be considered as well. If possible, you will also want to factor your parent's wishes into the equation.

If you're feeling confused about what to do, take a deep breath, then step back and look at the whole picture. Give yourself some time to gather as much information and input as you can. Find out how everyone involved in the decision feels about the situation. If there are conflicting opinions (and there very well may be), you'll need to figure out whose feelings you're going to have to prioritize at this point in time. What matters most to you? The stability of your marriage? Your children's lifestyle? Your parent's feelings? Your parent's health? The time and energy you already devote to your career or avocation? The opinions of the people in your social circle? There are no right or wrong answers here, so please don't judge yourself if you're unable to honor every single person's opinion or point of view. You can only do what you think is best once you've gotten all the information you can.

DESPAIR

In most of the stories we recount in this book, the adult child is dealing with only one living parent. The situation is different for Catherine, from Chapter 1, whose mother, Martha, had to undergo emergency hip replacement surgery. Her father, John, suffering from Parkinson's disease, now had to be cared for in a nursing home. Catherine's parents had grown very interdependent over the years, as they worked together to hide John's illness from the rest of the world. This made it very difficult for Catherine, who now had to try to make decisions that would please both her father and her mother, to say nothing of satisfying herself. Catherine's task could prove impossible. Trying to please everyone can result in despair, the sense that you can never get things quite right.

> Catherine accomplished a lot in the first few days after she received the phone call about her mother's accident. After visiting several nursing homes in the area to find a place for her father, she found St. Andrews. It was a small facility and was a little old-fashioned, but the staff was very friendly and Catherine had a good feeling about it. Catherine told herself that her father's placement was only for a short while. At first, John seemed very upset over the move. "I told him he'd only be there for a few weeks, until Mom got out of the hospital and recovered from her surgery," Catherine says. One of the best things about St. Andrews was its location near Catherine's home. She was able to visit her father every day on her way home from visiting her mother in the hospital.
>
> However, Martha didn't recover as soon as Catherine expected her to. She was diagnosed with severe osteoporosis. The doctor made it clear to Catherine that Martha needed help and would no longer be able to act as John's caregiver. Catherine thought this would probably be okay. After he'd

gotten settled in, John seemed happy enough at St. Andrews, and Martha would be able to visit him whenever she liked once she got out of the hospital.

For the next several weeks Catherine was torn between spending all her time with her mother at the hospital and her father at St. Andrews, and she was kept busy trying to make everyone happy. "It was exhausting," she says. "My mother was completely obsessed about things like whether the nurses had mixed exactly the right amount of cereal into Dad's yogurt. There was nothing I could do or say that would help her relax. If I told her that he seemed fine and looked comfortable to me, she said that he must be pretending. She needed to believe that it was impossible for him to live without her."

On one level, Martha knew she couldn't take care of John anymore, but on another level she believed no one else could do it just right. After she was released from the hospital, Martha made life difficult for anyone who had anything to do with her husband's care. She blamed Catherine for having chosen the "wrong" nursing home, she counted the pieces of underwear in her husband's drawer daily, she pushed the emergency button whenever no staff member was around, and, of course, she expressed adoration for her son, who lived overseas and who would never have made the same awful decision that Catherine had. "At first I felt proud of how well I had handled the whole situation," Catherine reports, "but after Mom got out of the hospital, I couldn't do anything right. It felt awful. I started to get angry whenever she complained about something. I even got a little jealous of my brother. He was in Germany and had no idea what was really going on, but Mom seemed to think he was the expert at everything. She insisted on calling him every few days to complain about something I had done. Sometimes I just wanted to strangle her!"

No matter what Catherine did, someone found it wrong. What was best for her father made her mother feel worthless and guilty. There wasn't any good solution at all, as far as Martha was concerned. And Catherine had yet to ask herself what was best for her. How could she even think of taking care of herself when she had so many other people to consider?

One of the most difficult emotional traps you can find yourself in is being torn between multiple solutions without an obvious "best choice." Not only can a dynamic like the one Catherine became embroiled in with her parents make you *feel* sick, but also it can actually make you physically ill from the detrimental effects increased stress has on your body. No matter what solution you choose, you will be hurting someone you love. Even the best logic can't save you from feeling awful in such a complex situation.

If you find yourself at the point of despair, consider stepping outside of the situation, if only for a day or two, to give yourself a clearer perspective on what is happening. Perhaps it would have benefited Catherine to take a few days off from visiting either parent or even from thinking much about the situation. Doing so might have helped her detach from everyone's demands, which would have helped her to think more clearly. In addition, during this challenging period be sure to boost your level of self-care above what you normally require. If you don't take good care of yourself, you won't be able to take care of anyone else for very long. Talk to someone you trust, and get some help and emotional support. You can't be all things to all people. It is simply impossible. Take care of yourself, and then do the best you can for everyone else involved. And remember to let your best be good enough.

HELPLESSNESS

Sometimes we desperately want to help someone because we believe he or she needs our assistance. When we offer help, if the person is not open to receiving it, we can end up feeling frustrated by a sense of helplessness. In the case of our parents, if they reject our help it can be particularly frustrating. In certain situations it is easy to think we know more about what is best for our parents than they do. This dynamic is the exact opposite of the idea most of us grew up with: that our parents know best. It can be difficult for our parents to accept the fact that perhaps the tables have turned and maybe they do need our help.

> Remember Amy from Chapter 2? Amy's first instinct after Ruth's wandering incident was to help her mother. But how? Ruth wouldn't even admit she had a problem. Amy spoke with doctors, social workers, and lawyers, who all told her the same thing. "Basically, they told me that as long as my mother's house was being cared for and Mom was coping okay with everyday life, there was nothing I could do," Amy says. "I told the doctor about my mom wandering off in the night, and she said there was nothing I could do to prevent it from happening again. My mother was an adult and she had a right to make care decisions for herself. But Mom didn't think she needed any help at all. It was really frustrating."

In that moment, Amy felt absolutely helpless. She was ready to do whatever her mother needed, and she even had her family's support, but her mother would not accept any help. As long as Ruth was legally able to make her own decisions, Amy could do nothing against Ruth's will. Ruth believed she was fine, so it was Amy who was under constant stress.

If you've ever been in a situation similar to Amy's you know how challenging it can be. You may want to consider asking a trusted relative, family friend, doctor, or clergy member to intervene with your parent on your behalf, but that may or may not work, depending on the person's relationship to your parent and his or her own assessment of the situation. If the person considers herself or himself a friend of your parent, she or he may not agree with you that your parent needs your help. If the person isn't close to your parent, his or her words are likely to fall on deaf ears.

Doctors can administer psychological tests to determine whether or not a patient is competent. However, it may be challenging to get your parent to take such a test, and you can't force him or her to do so. Furthermore, in some forms of dementia, such as Ruth's, the patient can go for long periods of time during which he or she is fully lucid and would be able to pass such a test—even if he or she had been off wandering the night before.

Depending on the laws in your area, you may be able to seek legal intervention by asking a doctor to declare your parent unfit, even against his or her will, and asking an attorney to put you in charge of your parent's affairs. Even if this is possible, think carefully before you do it. You may (or may not) succeed in gaining control over your parent's life, but you will undoubtedly damage or even destroy your relationship with your parent, probably forever. Before you take any action, spend the time needed to clarify for yourself what your own values and principles are, and how they are influencing your desire to help. You may not like doing nothing while your parent's abilities decline, but you may have to decide which is the lesser of the two evils. The truth is there is very little you can advisably do when a parent won't accept your help. In this type of situation, the task is to accept that you're simply unable to help your parent at the moment.

If your parent does not believe that he or she needs assistance, and you believe otherwise, we suggest that you read and practice the techniques described in the section on worrying. Your worrying won't change your parent's situation, but it can cause yours to deteriorate into a nightmare of stress and frustration.

HURT

A few weeks after her mother wandered off into the night, Amy got another strange phone call, this one from Ruth herself. "She was whispering like someone was listening," Amy tells us. "She said her neighbor had been stealing money from her. This neighbor was a woman we had known for years, and now Mom was saying that she had stolen more than eight hundred dollars!"

Amy wasn't sure what to do. She suggested her mother call the police. "She said she couldn't do that," Amy says. "She said the police were also stealing money from old people. She said I had to come over right away." Amy drove for an hour to Ruth's house. When she got there and asked her mother about the theft, Ruth had no idea what she was talking about. "She looked at me like I was the crazy one," Amy says. "She really thought I was the one who was losing my mind."

Over the next several months Amy received many strange phone calls from Ruth at all hours of the day and night. Ruth would whisper about some mysterious event or other, but when Amy arrived at Ruth's house she was always "back to normal." Whenever Amy or her husband, Mike, tried to speak directly with Ruth about the problem, she grew offended and angry and refused to discuss it with them. She began to accuse her daughter of plotting against her.

It took Amy more than a year to learn not to feel hurt about her mother's reproaches. She learned to take each new incident almost in stride. All she wanted now was to avoid losing contact with her mother altogether. She drove to her home to check on her almost daily. The day came when Ruth stopped letting Amy into the house, which was especially hard for Amy. Ruth thought Amy was stealing from her. Amy couldn't believe it; all she was trying to do was help, and now she was accused of stealing from her mother. But to Ruth, it all seemed perfectly logical. Why else would Amy be coming by so often now, when she had only shown up on Thanksgiving and Christmas for all those years?

It can be painful when we feel as though a parent is rejecting us. It can be difficult to remember that it is not the person rejecting us but rather the person's condition. Even though we understand that it is not "real" rejection, it still hurts.

You can't talk to an impaired person about your feelings. It won't work. If you are feeling hurt by your parent, it is important for you to get support and reassurance from someone else. Many cities have support groups for people who are in similar situations with their elderly parents. If you enjoy using the Internet, you may also find a number of good support communities online through a group site such as Yahoo or Google. (See the Resources in the back of this book for specific online group locations.) Whether in the "real" world or the online one, consider finding and joining a group of people who have some idea of what it's like to be in your shoes. If you can't find a group in your area, consider starting one. Yours is not an isolated problem. More people need this kind of support now than ever before.

WORRY

In most cases, something *will* happen some day. When you are suddenly responsible for the well-being of your parent or parents, you want them to be as happy and as healthy as possible, and you worry about what will happen if....

> Since there was nothing she could do to help Ruth, Amy began to worry about her. She began to imagine all sorts of terrible things happening to her mother. From the moment she received the phone call from the police officer, Amy faced tremendous changes in her life. She fretted about her mother constantly. She had trouble sleeping at night because she lay awake listening for the phone. She called Ruth's neighbors regularly to find out how her mother was doing. After Ruth stopped letting Amy into the house, Amy phoned her mother's neighbor twice a day. One day the neighbor told her that Ruth would not come to the kitchen door as usual. Amy raced to her mother's house and banged on the door.
>
> "She was in there," Amy recalls. "She yelled to me that she was fine. She said she was just lying on the sofa because it was so hot outside. But her voice was coming from the back of the house." Amy realized that her mother must have fallen, so she called an ambulance. The paramedic knocked on the door and called to Ruth. Ruth responded that everything was fine. "She told him to go away," Amy says. "When he asked her to please come to the door, she said she didn't have to. She kept saying that she knew her rights. Then she got really quiet. We had to break down the door to get inside."
>
> When Amy and the paramedics finally got inside, they found Ruth lying on the floor in the hallway outside the bathroom.

There may come a day when one or more of your worries become a reality. But only then will they truly be a reality. All the moments and hours and days and weeks you may have spent worrying in advance will not prevent it. Your worries only cause you extra grief and pain.

Worry is a tricky emotion because it feels productive. If you are worrying about someone, it can feel as though you're actually doing something for them. If we can't physically do something to help someone, we tell ourselves that we can do something emotionally. And so we worry.

Worry makes us feel miserable, and it makes us lose sleep. It weakens our immune systems and fills our bodies with toxic hormones, but in some odd way it also causes us to feel as though we are prepared for the worst. We may believe that worrying will make an event easier to deal with when it finally does happen. Of course, nothing could be further from the truth. Unless you have the psychic abilities to predict the future, there is no way to anticipate and prepare for every possible challenging event.

Some people may worry because it helps them feel as though they are taking the situation seriously enough. Others may do it just for show. People who don't worry about things are often portrayed as irresponsible or immature. The truth is, people who don't worry are probably much better prepared to handle the stress of a crisis than worriers are. Worry itself doesn't help anyone; it is only harmful. And it can easily become a bad habit. Worrying erodes the worrier's health and does absolutely nothing beneficial for his or her loved one.

The most difficult lesson to learn in certain parental-care situations is that for long periods of time you can do nothing. You must learn to be at peace with this fact. Worrying will only diminish your energy, energy you will need when something really does happen and you are called upon to act.

> "When Dad was living in our house," Pat, age fifty-nine, recalls, "his bedroom was across the hall from ours. I was always afraid he was going to fall down during the night. I would lie awake in bed just listening for him. In the mornings I was exhausted. One day my husband Peter woke up and found me still lying there worrying about Dad. 'Stop it!' he

shouted. He got really angry. 'You can't change anything by worrying! If he falls down, you'll hear it.' "

"I realized Peter was right," Pat says. "In all those years, Dad did fall three times. But we dealt with it each time, and I couldn't have prevented any of those falls by lying there awake and making myself sick with worry!"

Pat's husband got her to stop worrying by simply shouting at her in anger. But stopping worries is usually more than just a simple matter of willpower. If you're a worrier, try one or more of the techniques listed below to decrease your stress level. Or maybe you intuitively know other ways to help yourself stop worrying. Whatever it takes for you to stop worrying, please do it. Your worries are not productive in any way. Give yourself permission to release them and not to worry anymore.

Increase your level of physical exercise. Get your heart rate up and break a sweat. Do an aerobic activity that you enjoy, such as dancing, swimming, running, brisk walking, skating, or riding a bike. Unless your doctor advises otherwise, do something physical every day for at least thirty minutes. Exercise helps the body release toxins that build up when we worry, and it increases strength and energy levels. It also boosts the production of endorphins, the body's natural pain relievers and mood enhancers. Endorphins are responsible for the heightened sense of well-being that accompanies a good workout and that any regular exerciser can attest to. As a bonus, if you're doing something you enjoy, it will be easier to break the worry cycle while you're doing it, because your attention will be occupied elsewhere.

Make yourself a "fun and joy" list. Most worriers aren't having enough fun. List ten to twenty activities that bring you joy. They can be simple things, such as listening to a particular type of music, watching your favorite movie, or singing in the shower. Or maybe it's something more involved, like taking a trip to Disneyland. Once your list is complete for the moment (you can add to it at any time), display it where you can see it on a regular basis. Our friend Wendy hung her list on the refrigerator. Leslie, a client of

Lynn's, posted hers on the bathroom mirror. Resolve to choose at least one activity from your list each week and do it. Make time to have some fun and joy in your life.

Meditate or try guided visualization. Worry is negative mental chatter that makes us feel tense and edgy. It is mental noise that has emotional and physical effects. People who worry too much need to quiet their minds in order to break the cycle of worry. If you know how to meditate, try starting every day with some quiet time. If you don't know how to meditate or don't really want to, try purchasing a guided visualization audiotape or CD, such as one of those available for sale at www.lwnh.com (see Resources), and listening to it daily. A guided program will talk you through a cycle of relaxation designed to quiet your mind and help you gain more control over your thoughts. Think of meditation or guided visualization as a refreshing mental vacation from the stresses of worry and everyday life.

Try really catastrophizing! Psychologist Albert Ellis coined the term "catastrophizing" to describe a way of thinking that many people adopt when they worry. He suggested taking a really deep dive into your worries and asking yourself, "What's the worst thing that could possibly happen?" Come up with the most specific and most awful possibilities you can think of. Force yourself to get into your worries deeply, possibly even to the point of ridiculousness. Keep asking yourself, "Then what?" For example, "Mom could wander off and get lost and we'd never see her again and I'd never know what happened to her and she could starve on the street."

Most people find that when they get really clear about the worst thing they can think of, they realize one of three things: Either it isn't bad enough to warrant all the worrying, or it really is bad, but there is something that can be done to help (in the example above, putting an identification bracelet on Mom may help reduce worry). The third possibility is that you will realize worrying won't prevent your worst-case scenario. Sometimes just shining an imaginary light on a vague worry to make it more specific is all that is needed to help the worry evaporate into thin air.

Catastrophizing can be scary and even upsetting. If you happen to be in therapy already, consider asking your therapist to assist you in a catastrophizing session. You can also do it yourself with your journal and a pen, or just by talking it out with a supportive friend or clergy member. Remember that your goal is to get very clear about exactly what you are worried about and what role your worrying will play in preventing the situation.

Try the Serenity Prayer. If you find relief through prayer, try the famous Serenity Prayer, which has been used for decades by members of Alcoholics Anonymous. It is perfect for those who worry:

> *God, grant me the serenity to accept the things*
> *I cannot change,*
> *The courage to change the things I can,*
> *And the wisdom to know the difference.*

Try helping someone else. Much of our worry comes from being unable to help a loved one whom we perceive to be in need. But many other people are in great need of help and will eagerly and even appreciatively accept your assistance. Pitch in to help someone learn to read, feed the hungry in your town, volunteer at a senior citizen's center, rescue an animal, or clean up a local park. Whatever cause moves you, it can surely use your help. Spend your energy on something productive on behalf of someone else, and you'll be far less likely to spend it making yourself sick with worry about something you can't change.

ANGER

In almost every complex emotional situation, one or more of the people involved will feel angry at some point. Perhaps your mother is angry with you because you moved her into an assisted-living facility. Maybe your father is angry with you because you tried to discuss his finances with him. Your siblings may show anger when they try to figure out what to do about your parents' long-term care. And you may feel angry if it seems that no matter what decision you make you aren't going to be appreciated for it.

Although true anger demands expression and acknowledgement, anger can also act as a cover-up for more vulnerable and painful emotions. Be sure you understand what is beneath your anger before you yield to it. Are you really feeling unappreciated by your siblings for all the work you've done on behalf of your mother, but you can't say so? Are you feeling guilty about putting Dad in a nursing home against his wishes but don't want to admit that to him or to yourself? Do you resent all the time that caring for your parent is taking away from your life? If you can get a sense of what is really bothering you, you're halfway to releasing the anger that you feel.

When dealing with someone else's anger, it may help to understand that there's more going on in a temper tantrum than meets the eye. If your father rages at you for putting him in a nursing home, chances are underneath the anger he's feeling abandoned or rejected or vulnerable, or even all three, and is unable to express these feelings to you directly. If you know and understand this, his angry outbursts will be less hurtful and less likely to trigger your own anger. You can let him express his anger while you stay calm, knowing that it's not personal; it's simply about his feelings of loss.

True anger can be expressed in several ways, but for the expression of anger to be constructive it needs to be handled carefully. Most ways of expressing anger are harmful and can further damage an already fragile relationship. Yelling, screaming, name-calling, hitting things (or people), as well as passive-aggressive behaviors, such as ignoring others or agreeing to do something important and then not doing it, are all destructive ways of expressing anger. They will not ease the anger; they will only make matters worse for everyone else involved.

If you feel yourself needing to express your anger, choose to do it consciously and mindfully. Find a safe place to be alone, or get together with a person who will support you, such as a trained therapist, a clergy member, or a supportive friend. Then give yourself the gift of really feeling and expressing your anger. If you're alone, write furiously in a journal. Go ahead and write every angry, awful thought that comes into your head. Don't stop. Write until you feel completely drained of all anger, and then immediately destroy the paper and dispose of it. *Don't read it over* before you destroy it, or you'll just soak up all that anger again.

If you're with another person who has agreed to support you while you express your anger, allow yourself to say what you need to say. Cry, scream, hit a pillow, or do whatever you need to do to get the anger out. Ask the person you're with to hold a safe space for you and to let you express whatever you need to express. If you are angry at a specific person, it may help to imagine that person sitting in the room with you while you express your anger directly at him or her. Don't do this if the person you're angry with is actually present. Only do it in a room where he or she cannot hear you.

Once you've released your anger, you'll be in a better position to figure out what you need to change so you won't grow angry over the same situation again. Never confront a parent or sibling or other family member in anger. When you aim your anger at others, there is nothing they can do but defend themselves—perhaps by getting angry in return. Your message will not be heard, and your situation, rather than being improved, will be made worse. You must first get past the anger, then calmly approach the problem in a way that others are likely to be receptive to. For more strategies for addressing anger in family relationships, see the section in Chapter 10 on dealing with conflict between family members other than the nursing home resident.

DESIRE FOR REVENGE

We all have repressed emotions that we've judged as unacceptable because we didn't feel safe expressing or even acknowledging them when we first felt them. Those feelings are still inside of us. We may be unaware of them, but they impact our behavior. In the most extreme cases, they can cause us to nurse a deep-seated, probably unconscious, desire for revenge against someone, like a parent, who we believe somehow failed us. Take the case of Bert, who considered inviting his alcoholic father, Albert, to live with him and his wife, Susan. Bert was aware that he had never really gotten to know his father. He was conscious that he felt some urgency to spend time with his dad before it was too late.

Bert thinks he has forgiven his father. Indeed, his conscious intentions are only good-hearted. But can he be sure of himself? Does he really know what will happen the first time Albert fails to behave as expected? What will he do when his father becomes uncooperative (as he always has)? Will Bert be able to respond with patience when Albert is unreliable (as he always was), or when he lies to Bert (as he always did when Bert was younger)? Or is it possible that Bert harbors some unacknowledged—and thus unresolved—inner conflicts over Albert's alcoholism that could cause him to lash out toward Albert in a desire to punish him for old wrongs? These are important questions that Bert would need to consider if his father were to come and live with him and Susan.

Unresolved issues between parent and child can sometimes lead to abusive relationships based on the child's unconscious desire for revenge. Elder abuse is at an all-time high and is growing in frequency as our population ages. In 2000, according to a study by the National Center on Elder Abuse, nearly 170,000 cases were reported in the United States. Some experts believe that only about one in four cases gets reported, which would put the actual number of elder abuse cases at nearly 680,000 per year in the United States alone. Among states that collected data and reported it to the study, nearly 61 percent of all incidents of elder abuse took place in the home, and nearly 62 percent of those abused were harmed by a family member. By contrast, only 8 percent of reported instances of elder abuse took place in nursing homes. The number of nursing home incidences is far from perfect, but it equates to fewer than one in ten cases. Institutional caregivers ranked as perpetrators in only about 4 percent of all reported abuse cases. The widely divergent figures between home elder abuse and institutional elder abuse highlight the role that repressed emotions can play in a home-care situation.

If you find yourself in a situation where emotions such as resentment, anger, or desire for revenge are being expressed destructively toward others, do whatever you need to do to change the situation. This is true whether it is your emotions that are being expressed destructively or another person's. Hire more help, find a good therapist, put your parent in a good (or better) nursing home, and take better care of yourself. Do whatever it takes to release yourself from the destructive cycle of expressing negative, repressed emotions at the expense of another.

SHAME

"Go Away! Nothing is wrong!" Amy's mother Ruth insisted as she swatted at the paramedics who found her lying on the floor of her home. "It's my right to lie wherever I want! I'm going to sue all of you. My daughter is only trying to steal my money." Amy felt so ashamed.

In the hospital they discovered that Ruth had not washed her feet for months. Her toenails had grown so long that they had curled around and were cutting into the skin of her toes. Her feet were swollen, and she had an open sore that indicated possible serious problems with her circulation. "This is not a hospital case," the very young doctor told Amy. "This is a hygienic problem. You should look after your mother more carefully. Be sure her doctor treats that sore." Amy felt ashamed once more. She heard herself apologizing and trying to justify herself.

Ruth was in the hospital for two days. Whenever she saw Amy, she got very upset, but otherwise she didn't seem too unhappy. She seemed to enjoy the clean bed and even the shower.

Amy felt ashamed, helpless, and angry—all at the same time. No matter what she did, she felt there must be something she could be doing better. But there was nothing Amy could have done any better. Shame is a result of blaming ourselves for doing something "wrong." We may not even know what exactly we did. We just somehow feel we "should have" done better.

Some processes simply take time, including the development of problems associated with an elderly person's decline. Mental or physical function gradually weakens before a person is truly unable to live on his or her own. As time passes and you watch your parent's condition deteriorate, you may feel as though you know the inevitable outcome, so you want to do something right now. You may suffer from the uncomfortable sense that you are somehow failing. The truth is, when the time is right, the problem will become evident enough to require a solution. Until then, there's only so much you can do.

The territory of dealing with a parent's decline is new and unfamiliar to most of us. You are doing the best you can, even if you're not doing every single thing you can possibly think of. You are not to blame for your parent's condition, just as Amy was not responsible for Ruth's. Give yourself a break from judging yourself. Forgive yourself for anything you think you may not have done well enough. Try to see and accept the situation for what it is, not for what you think it should be, and allow yourself to release any shame you may be feeling. You simply don't need it.

LONELINESS

When you have to make decisions in a situation where communication with your loved one is no longer possible, you may feel utterly alone. When the pros and cons of a decision have been weighed and they come out even, or when you can't find any pros at all, it may be one of the loneliest times of your life. Just know that you are not wholly alone in all aspects of your life, that you can seek support when you need it, and that this too shall pass. If you feel the need for fellowship during this trying time, ask your doctor or the social worker at your parent's nursing home for a referral to a local support group or see Resources, at the end of this book, for information on some online support groups. In addition to offering support, members of an online group may be able to help you locate groups that meet in person in your area.

LOVE

Beth's reaction to the phone call she received about her mother's illness is probably what most of us would consider "normal." If you remember from Chapter 2, when Beth learned that her mother, Gwen, had suffered a stroke, she instantly dropped her plans for the future and began to imagine caring for Gwen at home.

> Beth's imagination failed to prepare her for what she found when she arrived at the hospital. "My first thought was that someone had made a mistake. There was no way this was my mother," says Beth. "She was so frail looking. Her face looked all twisted and ugly. She was frowning on one side of her mouth." That afternoon, Beth met with several nurses, an occupational therapist, a speech therapist, and a social worker. The friendly nurse's aide told Beth that her mother could no longer control her bladder and now had a catheter inserted. For her bowel movements Gwen wore incontinence pads, a larger version of children's diapers. Beth learned that her mother was going to need plenty of training and help with all her daily activities. She would be unable to go to the toilet alone, and it would take a long time for her to regain her speech, if it were possible at all. But at least she was alive.
>
> When Beth left the hospital nearly three hours later, she felt like an old woman herself. Was it just this morning that she was standing in her garden, full of energy and plans for the future? She felt thankful that her mother was still alive, but she also felt full of pity. How must her mother feel? Back home, Beth took a different look at her living room. This time her imagination didn't conjure an image of a wheelchair by the fireplace. She now pictured her mother's bed in the living room and an enormous tank for used diapers. She tried to envision how they would deal with the stairs.

Beth is in danger of taking on too much responsibility. She assumes she will bring her mother home because she thinks that is her duty as a good daughter. She wants to give back what she received from her mother when she was a child. Beth loves her mother, but her desire to provide home care is a first impulse. She hasn't reflected on the plan. Beth doesn't feel as though it would be a burden to take care of her mother. She knows it is what Gwen would expect, and she never even thinks about refusing.

Why, then, are we looking at Beth's situation? Isn't everything fine? Isn't it like a perfect mother-daughter storybook?

DEPENDENCY

The first sign of a problem is with the immediacy of Beth's reaction. She is not responding solely out of feelings of love and care, but also out of a spontaneous will to act, a need to change a situation. Beth doesn't bother to ask herself whether she is truly ready to bring her mother home. She never stops to consider whether it is a reasonable choice, given Gwen's condition after her stroke. It is difficult to tell if Beth's "yes" is a considered decision or simply the reaction of a (grown-up) child who doesn't dare to say no to her parent. It was Beth's daughter Kelly who first challenged Beth's decision.

> "When we spoke on the phone that night, Kelly told me not to do it," Beth remembers. "She told me her friend Kristen's family had their grandma at home after a stroke, and it was horrible. She said, 'Mom, it has nothing to do with love. The job is just way too hard.' She also said, 'You're a gardener, not a nurse!' That really shook me up. It was exactly what I didn't want to hear. She hit a button in me. I would have to give up my gardening plans."
>
> But what really upset Beth was when Kelly accused her of not having her own will. Kelly said to her mother, "You always do whatever Grandma wants you to!" Beth couldn't believe her ears. How could her eighteen-year-old baby say such a thing? Kelly seemed so sure of herself. So decisive.
>
> Beth didn't like what Kelly said, but she knew the truth when she heard it. She says, "When Kelly hit me with the uncomfortable truth, I knew she was right. I had always subordinated my will to my mother's. This time I couldn't give up my own life. I didn't like what I was hearing, but I decided to consider her heartfelt words an early Mother's Day present."

If you suspect that a pattern of dependency may exist between you and your parent, it is important to get help. It is very difficult to identify and break such a pattern when you're in the middle of it. You will need a supportive person who can see the dynamic between you and your parent from the outside. A good therapist, trusted clergy member, or supportive friend can assist you in identifying and breaking free from your old patterns and establishing some healthier new ones.

FEELING OVERWHELMED

Sometimes the responsibilities of caring for an elderly parent can seem overwhelming. There are so many things to do, so many decisions to make, and so many details to attend to. Whether you are caring for your parents in your home, helping them out as they stay in their own home, or moving them to another location, you have a lot to think about. There are bills to be paid and finances to be sorted out. There are possessions to be disposed of or to be repaired and maintained. There are caregivers to manage and other family members to keep updated. There are feelings to be shared. If all or even some of these responsibilities land on your plate in the midst of your own busy life, the situation can seem overwhelming. The good news is that there is a simple cure for feeling overwhelmed. By changing one small perception you can feel better almost instantly.

To release feelings of being overwhelmed, simply bring your mind into the now. If a large number of things need to be accomplished, just pick one and do it, without thinking about all the other ones. Take one step at a time, breathe, and stay focused on the present moment. Do only what you need to do *right now*, and you won't feel overwhelmed. It really is that simple.

If you continue to feel the need to imagine what is going to happen tomorrow or further down the road, at least choose to fantasize about positive things happening. You may think it's more "realistic" to imagine the worst, but the truth is you really don't know what will happen. If you're going to spend time thinking about the future, visualize things that are uplifting to you. Imagine yourself handling every detail perfectly. Imagine all your mother's or father's needs being met with grace and ease. Imagine everyone involved feeling happy and content with the situation. Who knows? It's quite possible that all your inspiring visualizations will have a positive impact on reality.

RELIEF

When a situation has been troubling us or making us feel stressed, and then it changes, we may feel some relief. But relief is often a mixed blessing. If our parent didn't want to go into the nursing home, our relief may be tinged with guilt. If someone we love has died, we may judge ourselves as wrong or uncaring for experiencing any feelings of relief. Relief is a normal and perfectly natural part of dealing with a stressful situation. If you feel relieved that a certain part of the situation is no longer your problem, enjoy the feeling. Avoid judging yourself as wrong or bad. Feeling relief simply means that one or more problems have been resolved and that you can now breathe a little easier.

GUILT

Guilt is a frequent companion of people who are responsible for a parent's care. If you put your mother in the finest nursing home in the city, but she complains about the food, you may feel guilty. If your sister takes Dad into her home after he has a stroke, you may feel guilty about not doing "your share." If you feel relief when your mother dies after a long illness, you may feel guilty.

The dictionary defines "guilt" as a combination of shame and regret over having committed a crime or done something wrong. But thanks to our early programming, many of us feel guilt when we haven't done anything wrong. When a loved one is unhappy with us for any reason, we often feel guilt. Even if that person's reason isn't justified, we may still feel guilty for "making" someone we care about unhappy. And if that someone is a parent who used guilt as a way to get us to behave when we were children, the weapon of guilt will probably work just as well today on our adult self.

The truth is, we don't make people happy or unhappy; that's a choice they make for themselves. We may choose the circumstances our parent is going to live in, but he or she will choose how to react to those circumstances. For every cranky, miserable person living in a nursing home, there are others in the same home who are cheerful, friendly, and delightful. Our circumstances don't determine our level of happiness; we do—and that goes for our parents, too.

Guilt doesn't help anyone. If your parents used guilt to motivate you as a child, you may find yourself instinctively using guilt on yourself, as though it will help you become a better person. But it doesn't work like that. If you like watching a certain television show, for example, you may feel guilty that you don't spend the time more productively. You'll watch the show, but you won't enjoy it. If you don't feel like visiting the nursing home one afternoon, you may feel guilty about it. You'll go anyway to avoid the guilt, but you'll have an awful time, and your parent will probably sense that you don't want to be there.

It is as if we somehow think that our guilt makes us better people. We seem to believe that if we allow ourselves to fully relax and enjoy our favorite TV show, we may become slothful and do nothing but watch television day and night for the rest of our lives. We fear that if we take a day off from visiting the nursing home without feeling guilty about it, we may enjoy ourselves so much that we never go back again.

Of course, the examples above, and others like them, sound foolish when we say them out loud. The truth is, if you let yourself enjoy your television show, you'll probably be refreshed and relaxed and ready to get busy when it ends. But if you beat yourself up for watching it the whole time you're sitting there, you're not going to feel like being productive when it's over; you'll be too exhausted from beating yourself up. If you take an afternoon off from visiting the nursing home and go enjoy a movie instead, you'll probably be much more ready to visit the next day. And if the movie was a good one, you'll have something interesting to talk about during your visit. But if you go to the movie and feel guilty while you're there, you won't feel like you got much out of the afternoon. You'll probably be too exhausted to visit the nursing home tomorrow.

Guilt is a kind of violence that we inflict upon ourselves. That's why we refer to feeling guilty as "beating ourselves up." If you consider yourself a peaceful person or one who doesn't condone violence, then release your guilt. You don't need it. It's not serving any useful purpose. Your guilt is not what makes you a good person. Let it go.

SADNESS

Regardless of how well your parent copes with aging or how well you cope with caring for your parent, some sadness may be inevitable. Let your sadness have its day. Cry all your tears and feel all your pain. Once it is fully felt and acknowledged, the sadness will pass and make room for you to smile again.

ANXIETY

Anxiety is a state of apprehension or uneasiness. It may be nameless and driven by vague worries or nervousness, or it may be more focused, such as the dread of discussing a specific topic. Life's little anxieties are completely normal. Deeper and more persistent anxiety needs to be looked at more closely. If you are experiencing frequent anxiety as you deal with your aging parent's needs, see your doctor as soon as possible. Get help before anxiety becomes a habit or a way of life for you—and possibly destroys your health.

RESENTMENT

If you are in a situation where you are required to take care of a parent and would rather be doing something else, you may experience some resentment, especially if your relationship with your parent has been, or has recently become, a challenging one. Much like feelings of aggressiveness or a desire for revenge, resentment is often thought of as an "unacceptable" emotion. We tend to tell ourselves it's not okay to feel resentful about taking care of someone who took care of us for so long. We believe it's not okay to resent helping someone whom we're "supposed" to honor and obey, so we repress those feelings. Consequently, resentment is one of the emotions that frequently gets pushed down and denied. And like its first cousin, the desire for revenge, repressed resentment can surface in harmful and abusive ways.

If you suspect that you may be resentful of your present circumstances, take a step back. Read the sections on anger and revenge in this chapter, and try some of the techniques described there to release and safely express your resentment. Then find a supportive group of people who can relate to what you're going through, and share your feelings with them on a regular basis. Resentment can eat you alive from the inside if you don't work to express and heal it in a safe and conscious manner. Healing and releasing resentment is an important part of taking care of yourself.

FEELINGS OF REJECTION

When you want to help but are rebuffed—or worse, accused of wanting to do harm—it's easy to feel rejected. Feelings of rejection are very common when our parents are old and decisions must be made about their care. Two kinds of rejection are especially relevant and worth mentioning here:

* Social rejection
* Parental rejection

Social rejection: You may have tried repeatedly to help your parent but have been met with refusal each time. That was Amy's situation with her mother. Amy wanted to help, but Ruth wouldn't allow it. Such circumstances can lead to a number of misunderstandings between you and outsiders. In Amy's case, for instance, she felt (mis)judged when the police officer said, "You should take better care of your mother," and when the young doctor told her, "This isn't a medical problem, it's a hygienic one. You should look after your mother more carefully."

The impressions of the police officer and the hospital staff are only the beginning. If you and your parents live or have lived in the same community, you may feel yourself becoming a target of gossip. You may lose some friends when they see your parent struggling and you "not helping." The good news about situations like these is that they will help you see who your real friends are. People who judge you or reject you socially on the basis of gossip are not your friends, and they are not contributing to your life in a positive and uplifting way. On the other hand, if you feel free to talk about your problems openly and honestly, you will deepen your relationships with people who respect and support you. When you are rejected socially over a misunderstanding like the kind Amy endured, your social circles will change—and these changes are likely to be for the better.

Feelings of social rejection can also take a slightly different form. Let's revisit Athena, from Chapter 4.

> When Athena's mother, Anne, decided to go into a nursing home instead of coming to live with her, Athena was wise enough to understand that what she thought was "right" might not have been right for her mother. But she still felt uncomfortable with the decision, because of her dependency on her social circle. "What will people think," she wondered, "when they find out my mother is going into a nursing home?" For a moment Athena considered hiding the truth. Her mother lived twelve hundred miles away—no one would know. But Athena was too smart to accept her own rationale.

Athena knows full well that people will know about her mother's care situation. What she doesn't yet realize is that if they are her friends, they *should* know. It will take some time before Athena is ready to tell them, and when she does she will find her social world changing. We're willing to bet that if Athena gives the truth a chance, those changes will be for the better.

Parental rejection: Feeling rejected by your own parent is one of the most difficult emotions to deal with. It's possible that Athena felt personally rejected by her mother's decision to live in a nursing home. After all, her mother rejected all the effort, time, and money Athena had already invested in helping her. Of course, Athena never actually asked her mother what kind of help she would have welcomed, so she was setting herself up for rejection by trying to make decisions for someone who was still capable of deciding for herself.

It was a different story for Aaliyah, the eldest of three middle-aged sisters. Aaliyah had felt used by her mother all her life. First, when her sisters were born it was Aaliyah who had to look after them. She always had to be the obedient big sister and set a good example. Then in her teenage years she had to hear that she had been born too early and had prevented her mother from having a career and leading her own life. Aaliyah had always tried hard to please her mother, but she never felt like she succeeded.

When her mother was old, it was Aaliyah who attended to all the daily details of her care. She managed the home-care staff and arranged for Meals on Wheels to deliver lunches. Consequently, Aaliyah felt desperately rejected and depressed when her mother decided to go live in a nursing home in another town, where Aaliyah's younger sister lived.

Many people go to great lengths to assist their aging parents, even to the extent of sacrificing their own dreams, health, and well-being. They often seem to think that their efforts will finally win them the approval they have always sought but never received. If you've been trying unsuccessfully for years to please your parent, please know that the situation isn't likely to change when Mom or Dad is at her or his weakest and most vulnerable. If your mom has withheld approval or your dad has been gruff and unforgiving, you can be pretty certain they are not going to give up those comfortably familiar behaviors now, when they are facing so much change and uncertainty.

Parental rejection can feel even worse if you find yourself losing your parent while he or she is still alive. When your parent suffers from some kind of dementia, as Amy's mother does, many aspects of your former relationship get lost. Perhaps your loved one no longer recognizes you. He or she has no smile, no thank you, no tenderness for you. Maybe he or she has become suspicious, anxious, or untruthful. You have lost your parent, one of the most important people in your life, while still taking care of him or her. If your parent were dead, you would have an opportunity to loosen the bond between you, to grieve in the "normal" way. But in cases of dementia, you are in the paradoxical situation of being the child of a parent who is now like your child. And when you suggest to Mom or Dad that she or he may need a little more help, you may be met with anger, denial, aggression, and rejection.

There is no cure for other people's rejection of us. We can't make others behave in a certain way just to make us more comfortable. The only place where we can deal with feelings of rejection is inside ourselves. If you are feeling rejected by another person you need to know that the rejection itself is not personal. It is not about you; it's about the other person. It is based entirely on the other person's needs, feelings, and perhaps misunderstandings and misjudgments about you. Sometimes that's just the way the world is. Don't take it personally. It may feel as though it's about you, but it's not. For some excellent and uplifting ideas about how to stop taking things personally, read *The Four Agreements*, by Don Miguel Ruiz. It's a small book that is very easy to read and understand, and it's very comforting. It may help you be more at peace with the situation that is leading you to feel rejected.

Emotional Soup

We've talked at length about your emotions and how they can impact your decisions about caring for your aging loved one. Sorting out one's emotions is difficult because they rarely pop up in isolation. They usually come in a combination of several, often contradictory feelings that seem to pull you in opposite directions. Your particular emotional mix will be unique to you and your situation, but it will almost always be the reason why you feel torn, confused, indecisive, or just plain frustrated. The exercise that follows will help you to more fully understand your emotional mix so you'll be better equipped to deal with the challenges of caring for an elderly loved one.

Exercise: Understanding Your Mix of Emotions

Once you know what you're feeling, it's a lot easier to deal with the various emotions and the issues they each present. Most professional therapists are experienced at helping people untangle complex webs of emotions. If you suspect that you're still dealing on some level with issues of childhood trauma or abuse, or if you simply feel stuck in an emotional quagmire, consider seeking help from someone who works in the emotional realm every day.

If you'd like to take a stab at untangling your own feelings, we've provided many questions to help you do so, organized into the following categories:

* Your actual situation

* Your feelings toward your aging loved one

* Your attitude toward sickness

* Your shared past with your aging loved one

* Your social environment

* Your attitude toward yourself

* Your attitude toward nursing homes

We suggest that you write out your answers. Writing allows you to uncover thoughts you may not otherwise have recognized, and it gives you an opportunity to review and reflect upon your responses later. The exercise may take a few hours or a few days to complete. Give yourself sufficient time. As you reflect on the issues raised here, you may find yourself making new observations about yourself, your parent, and other family members. You also will find yourself moving toward an understanding of your particular emotional mix.

YOUR ACTUAL SITUATION

What is urgent in your situation?

What is important?

Do you know the difference between the two?

Urgent things seem to need our attention right away, but important things are often overlooked until they become urgent. A ringing phone may seem urgent—"Answer me now!" it seems to say—but it may not be important. Getting your mother to see the foot doctor may not seem urgent, but it is probably more important than it seems. Don't wait for important things to become urgent before you attend to them.

Who is pushing you?

What can wait until later?

What can be done by others?

What services can be bought?

Who owes you a favor that you can call in now?

YOUR FEELINGS TOWARD YOUR AGING LOVED ONE

You feel love. Do you feel anything else?

Have you ever felt dominated or oppressed by this person?

Have you developed a dependency on him or her?

Have you been disappointed by this person?

Has this person ever abused you?

Have you ever felt used or unappreciated by this person?

Are you under pressure from this person or others in your life to follow a certain course of action you may not want to take?

Have you ever borrowed money from this person, causing you to feel obligated to pay him or her back somehow?

Do your best to uncover the emotional patterns and various "scripts" that are running inside your head and heart about this person. This may well be the most complex aspect of your assortment of emotions. Don't expect the revelations to end when you finish reading this chapter. If you keep searching inside, you'll discover new things about your feelings for this person for a long time to come.

YOUR ATTITUDE TOWARD SICKNESS

What are your experiences with sickness and disabilities in general?

What are your feelings about them?

How do you feel when you see a stranger in a wheelchair?

Can you relate to the person at all? Or do you prefer to look away?

If you tend to look away from people with disabilities, don't feel bad about it. Do your best to gently bring yourself around to getting to know one or more disabled people. After spending some time with a handicapped person, you may see that his or her disability seems to fold almost invisibly into the fabric of his or her life. The human organism is capable of making huge adjustments. Even people who suffer enormous physical difficulties simply develop a new kind of "normal" life. It is still the same person inside the damaged body. The late actor Christopher Reeve, who was paralyzed for the last ten years of his life from a horseback-riding accident, served as an inspiring example of what disabled people are capable of accomplishing.

If you have a very hard time looking at the sick and disabled, you may have what Xenia calls an acute aesthetic sensitivity. If your idea of beauty tends to emphasize things that are in harmony, especially visual harmony, it may be impossible for you to develop a true comfort with the uglier aspects of sickness or misery. If this seems to describe you, don't try to hide your sensitivity. Sooner or later the sick person will become aware of how you feel and may be offended. When someone is sick, his or her senses are very open to these types of energies. So it's a good idea to be honest. Avoid visiting your loved one when you know it's bedtime and he or she is lying in bed without his or her teeth. Instead, go at tea time, or when uplifting events are scheduled. You don't have to be ashamed of your sensitivity; just be honest about it. You can talk about it delicately and kindly and without going into too much detail, for example, "Mom, I'm sorry, but it just upsets me to see you without your teeth. But I want to visit you a lot, so I'm going to try to time my visits to coincide with your recreation hour." Don't try to explain too much about your sensitivity to many people. Those who feel differently may not understand and may even judge you. Those who feel the same way you do will understand plenty without your having to use any words at all.

YOUR SHARED PAST WITH YOUR AGING LOVED ONE

What was your relationship with your loved one like when you were younger?

Are there any special traditions and events you remember sharing together?

Are there any specific painful memories that come up? Were you well treated in general?

If circumstances permit, consider asking your loved one to share with you any special memories he or she may have of your previous life together.

As you write your answers to these questions, be prepared for a lot of memories connected with your loved one to come up. For the first time in years, you may recall your first love, your first puppy, or your first car accident. Your memories may be very tender and pleasant, or very harsh and cruel. No matter what comes up, welcome the feelings that come with it. Long-repressed painful or difficult emotions may be crying out to be expressed and healed. Your loved one's past is partly your past, and this can make for a complicated situation. Just accept the memories as they arise, and feel the feelings associated with them. Every memory connected to a feeling affords you an opportunity to keep moving forward by looking back.

YOUR SOCIAL ENVIRONMENT

Who do you feel is watching you?

Whose opinion is important to you? That of your colleagues at work? That of your other community members (religious, academic, social)? That of certain relatives?

In what areas of your life do you feel it is important to make a "good impression"?

How much power over yourself do you give these people?

How dependent are you upon them or upon their good opinion of you?

Is there anyone in your family or wider social circle whose opinion you regard as more important than your own?

This area may be an uncomfortable one to explore. You may find it difficult at first to be truly honest when answering these questions, but it is very important to become conscious of what is driving you to act the way you do. Understanding the role that your social environment plays in your behavior can be very liberating in the long run.

YOUR ATTITUDE TOWARD YOURSELF

In what ways are you strict with yourself?

In what ways are you permissive with yourself?

Do you tend to invest too much energy in unimportant projects?

Are you currently withdrawing too much from your energy "bank account"?

Do you sometimes say yes when you'd rather say no?

Are you comfortable setting boundaries and sticking to them?

Are you a "good" son or daughter?

What are some of the ways in which you take care of yourself?

YOUR ATTITUDE TOWARD NURSING HOMES

What have you heard about nursing homes?

How do your friends talk about nursing homes?

How do the media in your area portray nursing home life?

Do you have firsthand experience with a nursing home?

Has your parent ever expressed a desire "never to be put away" in a nursing home?

Have you heard that nursing homes are ugly, disgusting places filled with cruelty and abuse?

You already know that dealing with the care of your elderly parent is a challenging and complex emotional situation, made trickier by all kinds of social and familial factors, many of which are beyond your control. Whether or not you're not a fan of nursing homes at this point, do read on. Part II of the book will show you some interesting and valuable things about today's much misunderstood nursing home. The information you gain will help you clarify and resolve your situation.

You've Decided…
Now What?

Chapter 6
Finding the Right Nursing Home

Chapter 7
Once You've Found a Facility You Like

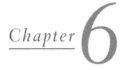

Chapter 6

Finding the
Right Nursing Home

As we said in the Introduction, once you've made the decision to move your parent or loved one into long-term care—or your parent has made this decision for himself or herself—you're ready for this part of the book. This chapter introduces you to various types of long-term-care facilities and helps you determine which one is best for your particular situation. It also offers a variety of useful tips and a comprehensive checklist for determining whether the quality of the facilities you are considering meets your standards.

In this chapter we also give you guidelines on what to look for in a nursing home, both the good and the not so good, so you'll be confident that the facility you choose is one you can trust. The next chapter discusses the steps to take once you've settled on a particular facility.

Of course, you can also read this part of the book if you're still making the decision about long-term care. Understanding some of the details about what distinguishes different facilities from each other can be a useful and reassuring tool in the decision-making process. We believe that after reading this material you'll see that there's a facility out there that your loved one can be happy *in* and you can be happy *with*.

A Change in Abilities Calls for a Change in Living Arrangements

Before we describe the different kinds of nursing homes, let's start with something even more basic: How can you know when your elderly parent is ready for a particular living arrangement? Is there a checklist for each category of long-term-care facility? Not exactly, but here we offer some guidelines based on quality-of-life issues that you can observe in your aging loved one and probably also can relate to based on your own experiences.

Adults go through different life stages that are characterized by changes in their abilities and desires. In the period sometimes called the prime of life, you have a feeling that you can accomplish anything you want to. You enjoy reasonably good health, and you have the energy to travel if you wish. You have enough time and money to pursue your interests, and you take pleasure in your family and friends. If your parents are feeling this way, there is no need to consider moving them into any kind of long-term-care facility at this time. You may disagree with their assessment of their abilities, but there is little or nothing you can do about it, so relax and let them enjoy life.

At other times you feel tied to your community. You value friendly neighbors and the security that comes from being part of a structured community. You enjoy a relatively fixed routine each day. Your parent or parents may still feel this way, or they may not. Perhaps their needs for community are no longer being met where they currently live. Maybe your mother is the only senior citizen left in a neighborhood filled with young families, and she doesn't feel a part of the gang anymore. Perhaps most of your parents' friends have moved away. If this is the case and your parent or parents are still healthy and want to take part in an active community of people with whom they are likely to have much in common, it may be time for them to consider making the move to a dedicated retirement community.

Maybe your parent or parents are at a time in their life when they really don't want to leave the house. It's enough just to deal with everything that's going on within their own four walls. Your mother or father may like to keep the place in order, but it's starting to become a bit of a burden. If you sense that your parent or other elderly loved one is beginning to feel this way, it may be time to consider helping him or her make the move to an assisted-living facility.

There may even come a time when your parent or parents don't want to leave their bedroom. For a moment, imagine yourself in their situation. Everything outside is a burden. It is a major effort to go to the bathroom or even to walk the five feet from the chair to the window. Your legs hurt, and every breath reminds you of your weak heart and nagging respiratory problems. Your world has a radius of about eight feet around you. If your parent is feeling this way, you may want to begin talking with him or her about making the move to a nursing home.

Finally, imagine there comes a time when you feel exhausted just sitting up in bed. This feeling can happen to anyone at any age—perhaps after surgery or while in the hospital during an illness. After two hours of sitting in a chair, you want to take a little nap. You can no longer take care of yourself, even in the bathroom. What you probably enjoy most is the feeling that skilled, caring people are there to support you when you need them. At mealtime they lead your hand to your mouth without making you feel like a child. In the bathroom they assist you without making you feel ashamed. They help you wash yourself without making you feel naked, exposed, or vulnerable. If your parent is in this situation, it's time to find a good nursing home.

Different Kinds of Long-Term-Care Facilities

When it comes to helping the elderly on a day-to-day basis, a number of options exist (besides home care). One or more of them may be right for your parent. Although different sources may refer to these facilities by different names, we have tried to use the most common terminology.

The following are the general categories of long-term-care facility:

* ✽ Group homes for the elderly
* ✽ Board-and-care facilities or rest homes
* ✽ Retirement communities
* ✽ Assisted-living facilities
* ✽ Rehabilitation centers
* ✽ Skilled nursing homes
* ✽ Specialized Alzheimer's and other dementia units

In this section we briefly describe each and highlight some of their advantages and disadvantages. After reviewing this material, you'll be able to weigh each option against your situation, taking into account your loved one's condition and preferences as well as what types of facilities are available in your area.

Within each category, other differences exist, too, which cannot be listed and described quite as easily. These differences can be thought of as sort of a nursing home microcosm of the American melting pot. If you traveled through America you could encounter a multitude of cultures; various ethnic and social groups; dozens of languages; myriad customs, religious practices, and rituals; and numerous types of dwellings, large and small. You would pass through many neighborhoods, some very poor, filled with people who work hard and are just getting by; others quite affluent; some unsavory or filled with tension; others peaceful and harmonious. If you traveled the same route from nursing home to nursing home, you would observe the same differences.

GROUP HOMES FOR THE ELDERLY

Group homes aim for the residents to live in as normal a household environment as possible, with assistance from each other. In the United States, group homes are more commonly designed as residences for disabled people and for people who are in recovery from various addictions. However, across Europe and in some U.S. cities, group homes also exist for the elderly. Group homes for the elderly usually require residents to be mobile when they move in, but they needn't be of sound mind. The home has a caregiver on staff who strives to get everyone involved in the activities of community living; the goal is often to approximate a family environment. For example, everyone may pitch in to the best of his or her ability to make and serve dinner and clean up afterwards.

The environment in a group home can be very warm and loving, but it can also be romanticized or idealized by the family members of residents. Sometimes certain residents aren't interested in bonding or "playing house" with each other. Occasionally, organizational problems crop up in group homes that would be lessened by the systems in place in a larger facility. For example, group homes often have only one caregiver on duty at a time. This can be a problem if the caregiver is helping one resident on the toilet while another is in need of urgent attention.

BOARD-AND-CARE FACILITIES OR REST HOMES

Before about the 1960s, people would typically go to live in a rest home when they got old and could no longer drive, manage the stairs, do their own shopping, or get dressed by themselves. Rest homes were large residences that rented out rooms to older people and assisted them as needed with some of the basic activities of daily living. Since they were often located in smaller towns and populated with the town elders, rest homes didn't usually have the stigma attached to them that nursing homes do today. The rest home of yesteryear has evolved into the board-and-care facility of today. It's a familial environment, somewhat like a hotel, but with more care and attention paid to the residents depending upon their needs and personalities.

The level of quality at any board-and-care facility depends on the owner. Just as there are low-quality and low-budget hotels, there are low-quality board-and-care centers, and there are others that are absolutely wonderful. If you're looking at a board-and-care facility, ask what kind of care is provided by the owner and what his or her particular qualifications and experience are. Often, the owner is strictly an administrator who hires qualified staff members to care for the residents.

RETIREMENT COMMUNITIES

Retirement communities are designed for healthy, active retirees who want to live in a secure and mature environment. Often the facility offers organized leisure activities, but the residents own their own homes or rent their own apartments within the community and can come and go as they please. Although retirement communities themselves are not considered a form of long-term care, many offer long-term-care units on site. Some may even have their own doctors or be affiliated with hospitals. These arrangements allow residents to move in when they are still healthy and stay for life by adding different levels of assistance, such as meal plans, when it becomes necessary.

ASSISTED LIVING

In an assisted-living facility, residents live in apartments or suites of their own, which they can rent furnished or unfurnished. Just like in the "real" world, the apartments in an assisted-living facility may be small studio apartments or larger units with one, two, or three bedrooms. Some assisted-living facilities allow residents to purchase extra services. They may opt in or out of meal plans, housekeeping, twenty-four-hour care, transportation, and other amenities. In other facilities, all services are included in one set price, whether or not the resident wants to take advantage of those particular amenities.

An advantage afforded by some assisted-living arrangements is that care can be provided by a combination of family members and staff, depending on the schedules and lifestyles of the resident's relatives. Family members can be "on duty" during certain hours, and the staff of the facility can fill in for them the rest of the time.

It is best for residents of assisted-living facilities to be of sound mind and to be able to make rational decisions for themselves. In an assisted-living apartment, you have the same rights as if you were renting an apartment in any building. No one may enter your apartment against your will, you may entertain guests, and you have the right to get as dirty as you like and not take your medication if that's what you choose. No one "controls" the residents of an assisted-living facility against their will.

Some assisted-living facilities have special sections for residents with Alzheimer's disease and other forms of dementia. These areas are not really part of the assisted-living arrangement, but if a resident has lived independently for some time, there is less stigma and trauma if he or she only has to move down the hall or into the next building for care. In this way, the resident can remain a part of the larger community she or he has become accustomed to.

REHABILITATION CENTERS

A rehabilitation center is similar to a nursing home, but it is designed for short-term stays. Rehab centers only accept people with certain conditions that could potentially improve. Residents are usually admitted after a hospital stay and with a doctor's referral. To receive benefit from rehabilitative care, residents must be willing and able to attend therapy sessions designed to help them regain some abilities. Your parent may want to enter a rehabilitation center if he or she has suffered a very mild stroke and has potential for recovery with training, if he or she has undergone joint-replacement surgery and needs care for a few weeks or months while healing, or if he or she has had a heart attack and can't live alone until regaining some strength.

NURSING HOMES

Sometimes called convalescent homes, nursing homes are more than just places to live; they also supply skilled medical care and ongoing medical observation. People often consider nursing home placement before it is truly necessary—when assisted living or a retirement community may be more appropriate.

To help you determine whether it is time for your parent to go into a nursing home, find out how your parent feels about the place where he or she is living now. As a simple rule of thumb, if your mother or father feels overly sad or wistful about leaving and can still manage most day-to-day activities, it is probably not yet time to move to a nursing home. It is time to make the move to a nursing home when your loved one feels burdened by his or her possessions and by the responsibilities of maintaining a household and desires some relief. Of course, most situations aren't as clear-cut as being sad one day and being ready to leave for the nursing home the next. Your parent is likely to have a number of mixed feelings at any given time, but using the general guidelines described here should help keep most families from overcomplicating the matter.

> Xenia's mother, Maria, had never seen the inside of any nursing home, even the facilities that her daughter owned—but she had vowed never to live in one. Maria lived alone in an apartment. As she got older she pretty much isolated herself. One day, she fell and injured herself and was taken to the hospital. When it was time to leave the hospital, Xenia took Maria into one of her nursing homes to recover. Maria was angry and vowed to return to her own apartment as soon as possible.
>
> After three months in the nursing home, Maria was able to go home. She left in a huff and headed back to her own place. Three weeks later Maria called Xenia and asked sweetly if she could come back to the nursing home to live for good. She said, "It's easier to look for my glasses in one room than it is in three!"

SPECIALIZED ALZHEIMER'S (AND OTHER FORMS OF DEMENTIA) UNITS

Although many nursing homes accept dementia patients, some facilities are designed specifically to deal with the special needs of this group. These homes strive to maintain more of a connection to the residents' former lives than other types of facilities do. They engage residents in reminiscing and use special older-style furnishings to jog memories. The environment is secure and safe so residents can wander around. Staff members communicate with residents at their ability levels, for example repeating themselves as necessary for those who need it. Staff members are trained to meet the mental, physical, emotional, social, safety, and friendship needs of dementia patients.

What Kind of Care Does My Parent Need?

The chart on pages 127 and 128 will assist you in evaluating the best type of placement for your parent or other loved one. First, from the left-hand column choose the description or descriptions that most accurately describe your loved one's condition or abilities. For each one of these selections, the check marks in the corresponding row will indicate which type(s) of facilities are best suited to meet your loved one's needs. You can circle the check marks that apply and make a tally of them by column to see which type or types of facilities you should consider most carefully.

We have intentionally *not* included check marks under the headings for board-and-care homes and group homes because each one is unique and will have its own requirements. For example, some may provide basic nursing services and others may not; some may accept dementia patients and others may not. If there is a board-and-care facility or group home for the elderly near you, pay it a visit with this checklist in hand to determine whether or not the fit makes sense in your situation.

Once you have a sense of what type of facility your parent's condition calls for, you are ready to proceed to the next step: choosing a specific home. Ultimately, this decision will depend on several other factors in addition to the type of facility your parent requires. We'll discuss these factors in the rest of the chapter, and you will be able to apply them to your unique situation to make the best decision for you and your loved one.

Note that for simplicity, as pointed out in Chapter 1, we'll continue to use the term "nursing home" generically to mean any type

What Kind of Facility Is Best for My Loved One?

MY PARENT…

	Assisted living	Retirement community	Short-term rehab center	Nursing home	Dementia unit (Alzheimer's, etc.)	Board-and-care home	Group home
1. … can drive a car safely.	✓						
2. … is strongly impaired in both sight and hearing.				✓			
3. … would be able to learn how to drive a golf cart.	✓	✓	✓				
4. … is full of plans and is able to execute them.	✓	✓					
5. … could still do many things if only he/she were more motivated.	✓		✓				
6. … enjoys playing an active role in the community.	✓	✓					
7. … needs some support with washing him-/herself and dressing properly.	✓						
8. … needs total support with personal care.			✓	✓	✓		
9. … can physically do personal care but needs general supervision and motivation.	✓		✓	✓	✓		
10. … can physically do personal care but needs total supervision.					✓		

From *Living Well in a Nursing Home* … Copyright © 2006 by Lynn Dickinson & Xenia Vosen, Ph.D. Order from Hunter House Publishers. (800) 266-5592

What Kind of Facility Is Best for My Loved One? (Cont'd.)

MY PARENT...	Assisted living	Retirement community	Short-term rehab center	Nursing home	Dementia unit (Alzheimer's, etc.)	Board-and-care home	Group home
11. ... would not cook anything for him-/herself if not supervised.	✓				✓		
12. ... cannot organize his/her plans for the next day.					✓		
13. ... is more than temporarily disoriented.					✓		
14. ... has experienced some sudden physical deterioration.			✓	✓			
15. ... has no incontinence problems at all.	✓	✓					
16. ... can handle eventual incontinence problems him-/herself.	✓	✓	✓				
17. ... needs some physical assistance with his/her incontinence problems.	✓		✓	✓	✓		
18. ... needs total support with his/her incontinence problems.			✓	✓	✓		
19. ... has some physical problems but is able to ask for help and is cooperative about receiving it.	✓						
20. ... is willing and able to invest energy to improve his/her physical situation.			✓				

of long-term-care facility. The factors that go into making your decision apply to each of the categories of long-term-care facility described above. Don't worry if your parent isn't currently in need of a nursing home specifically. The rest of this chapter and the next few will still be very helpful to you.

Beginning the Search

All long-term-care facilities have certain things in common that are easy to evaluate. Once you know what they are you will be more prepared to decide whether a certain place will or will not work for your mother or father. Reading the rest of this chapter will help you know when you have found a good nursing home and when to walk away and keep looking.

The first steps are to find nursing homes and evaluate them according to—

* location

* size

* ownership/culture

* your financial situation

* facilities and services offered

* nursing home staff

The next several sections of this chapter examine each of these criteria in detail.

Location: Finding Nursing Homes in Your (or Your Parent's) Area

There are several ways to locate nursing homes and other long-term-care facilities in your area:

* Contact your local or state council on aging.

* Browse through the yellow pages.

✳ Use the Internet. Online services such as MyZiva.net are available to help locate nursing homes in different geographic regions. MyZiva.net bills itself as "the complete nursing home guide" (see Resources). It offers detailed information about specific nursing homes, including comparisons with other facilities in the same county. Some information services are funded by the nursing homes themselves, and some by the professionals and advertisers that use them.

Once you have a list of facilities in your area, contact them to learn more. Most nursing homes will happily mail you a brochure and other material. Those with websites may provide "virtual" tours. Perusing the material provided by the nursing home can provide you with enough information to rule out some of the facilities on the basis of your preferred size, cost, philosophy, or culture.

The next step is to call the facilities you are still considering and ask to speak with the person in charge of admissions. You may want to have the checklist from this chapter in front of you when you call, to guide your conversation and remind you of questions to ask. This screening may help you to rule out one or more nursing homes based on their answers to your questions and the way the admissions officer interacts with you on the phone. If you are not well treated when you call, take note; this is an important piece of information.

After you narrow down your list, you may have one or more facilities in mind that you wish to visit. If neighbors or friends have had personal experience with any of these homes, now is the time to ask their opinions. Be sure to listen closely to what they say regarding their feelings about the facility while remaining open to making up your own mind about it. Every person's experience is different, just as every person's care needs, personality, preferences, and health situation are different.

Two important points to consider when evaluating the location of a nursing home are the following:

* Whether you want an urban or a rural environment

* The proximity of the nursing home to you

URBAN OR RURAL?

Maybe your parent or other loved one is very attuned to nature and would thrive if they had a beautiful ocean view or woodsy surroundings. If this is the case, by all means prioritize your nursing home brochures based on the gardens surrounding the buildings or the views from the rooms. On the other hand, if your parent is visually impaired or hearing impaired, he or she may not need a lovely view or pastoral setting.

Be careful to avoid choosing your parent's surroundings just because they look peaceful and relaxing to you. If you have a busy life it may be tempting to choose a calm atmosphere for your parent, but if you had to live in that environment for weeks, months, or years, you might find it very dull indeed. Many people find nature settings far less interesting and stimulating than city life. Even people who have lived their whole lives in the country may find an urban environment more engaging now that they are taking a more passive role. Many older people love to spend their time sitting and looking out the window at the everyday comings and goings. Fire engines, police sirens, even traffic moving in and out of the parking lot are all of interest to many nursing home residents. No matter how beautiful the view is, if the scenery never varies, it could get boring very quickly. The reverse may be true as well. A lifelong city dweller may be ready for the peace and quiet afforded by living in the country.

The point we're making is to be sure to provide your parent with the environment that he or she will find the most stimulating. Sometimes the only way to know for sure whether you've chosen well is to give the facility a try. It may be difficult for your parent to imagine being happy in a place that is at first so foreign, but you may be surprised by how quickly your parent becomes engaged in an environment that he or she finds new and exciting.

PROXIMITY TO YOU

How close should your parent's nursing home be to where you live? In most cases, moving your parents closer to you means taking them out of the environment they have lived in for many years. If your parents are still aware of where they are, or if they still have friends in their home community, it may be best to find a home near where they are already living. Although it can hurt to think that your mother or father may prefer to live near friends rather than close to you, you can probably imagine how you would feel if the situation were reversed.

Another thing to consider is how fast your parents' neighborhood is changing. If the place where they live hasn't changed in decades, they may feel most comfortable there. On the other hand, if new buildings are going up on every corner and the area is developing rapidly, they may not recognize their neighborhood in a few years and may be willing to move into a nursing home closer to where you live.

One more factor is your relationship with your parent. If you plan to visit frequently, you'll want your parent nearby, but please read the section in Chapter 9 on how often to visit before you make that decision. Adult children of nursing home residents often feel they would be doing the best thing for their parent if they were to visit every day, but often this is not the case. Besides reading Chapter 9, take a realistic look at your schedule, your lifestyle, and your past relationship with your parent. Doing so can give you a better sense of whether the urge to visit frequently is really a good enough reason to move your parent into a nursing home closer to where you live.

Size of the Nursing Home

In general, nursing homes come in the following four sizes:

1. Extra small or "micro"
2. Small

3. Medium

4. Large

EXTRA-SMALL NURSING HOMES

Micro-sized or extra-small nursing homes are those licensed to care for up to twelve residents. They are more like a family home than an institution and in most cases are run by an owner and his or her family. Extra-small nursing homes can be wonderful, warm, inviting places where you feel at home and relaxed the minute you walk in the door. Yet the small size also presents certain dangers because the facility is more like a home-care situation than a nursing home in terms of the number of caregivers and the daily schedule. Extra-small nursing homes usually cannot afford to offer a lot of activities or to hire a large, well-trained staff. The owner/director often lives on site and is "on call" night and day. Sometimes this can lead to exhaustion and extreme stress, in the same way that a home-care situation can. It can also lead to insufficient care of the residents or slow response time in situations of urgency. If multiple residents need to use the bathroom at the same time that a resident with dementia is getting into the medicine cabinet, an emergency can result and overwhelm the small staff.

Elderly residents sometimes stumble and fall. They occasionally pull the tubes from their own or another's respirator, or they may not realize that the knife they are holding is very sharp. If your parent needs only minimal supervision and assistance, a very small nursing home that you feel good about may be just the place. But if your loved one needs regular attention, be sure to find out if the micro-sized nursing home you are considering can confidently take on his or her care.

SMALL NURSING HOMES

Small nursing homes are those licensed to care for about twelve to forty residents. They are an ideal size for many people—small enough to offer a homey feeling, but large enough to be run in a professional manner. You may like knowing all the staff members, and your parent may enjoy the stimulating environment afforded by a slightly larger facility.

Small nursing homes often have financial problems. One or two empty beds or a couple of residents who fail to pay on time may represent a loss of 10 percent or more of their income, which can be quite significant in the low-profit-margin world of nursing homes. Ask direct questions to make sure that any difficult financial situations are dealt with by the owner's taking less profit or implementing cost-cutting measures that don't affect the overall quality of care, rather than by reducing important services to residents. It is probably fine if laundry service is reduced to every other day to save money, but if the home cuts its staff, stay alert to changes in the quality of your parent's care. It is not unheard of for an unscrupulous nursing home to sedate residents to make them easier to care for, or to use catheters at night instead of paying an aide to take them to the bathroom. Of course, if the staff is reduced because of empty beds, the staff-to-patient ratio may remain at an acceptable level and your parent's care may not be compromised. Simply pay attention, and be sure to ask some direct questions if you hear of cost-cutting measures being implemented at your mother's or father's nursing home.

To be sure, cost cutting is a fact of life in most institutions around the country, not only at nursing homes. Schools, hospitals, and many other organizations, both publicly and privately funded, have faced the need to cut costs at one time or another. Nor is the problem of reduced services unique to small nursing homes. Larger facilities may reduce services to increase the owner's profit, and even nonprofit homes are not above cutting costs by reducing services. We mention this particular risk here, in the section about small homes, because whenever they have empty beds they are in more danger of suffering financial problems than large homes are.

MEDIUM-SIZED NURSING HOMES

A medium-sized nursing home is licensed to care for approximately 40 to 120 residents. Medium-sized homes are usually separated into units, each of which houses roughly 18 to 25 residents and has its own staff and team leader. Medium-sized nursing homes have a well-developed management system devoted to each group of tasks: food preparation, housekeeping, nursing and resident care, and administration and management.

A medium-sized home will likely be run more systematically and professionally than a small one, but it may afford less one-on-one communication with the director or other staff members. Medium-sized facilities may offer a less familial atmosphere than smaller ones; consequently, it may take a new resident longer to adjust to his or her surroundings.

LARGE NURSING HOMES

A large nursing home is licensed to care for more than 120 or 150 residents. Some have more than 400 residents. Large homes can sometimes offer residents lower monthly fees because they are usually able to reduce operating costs by centralizing services and purchasing supplies in bulk. They have other advantages as well. They may provide more extensive options for therapy and a community that is more diverse and compatible with your parent's needs. A small or medium-sized nursing home, for example, may have only one or two residents with Parkinson's disease, and while the home may be able to care for those residents quite well, perhaps it is unable to offer special therapies for Parkinson's. By contrast, a large nursing home may have twenty or thirty residents with the disease, providing a new resident who has Parkinson's both with a built-in community of others who understand what he or she is going through and possibly also with specialized group activities and therapies designed for Parkinson's patients. Large nursing homes can offer their employees more development and training opportunities. They may provide tuition-reimbursement benefits or regular on-site training sessions to keep the staff up to date on the latest techniques, standards, and findings in resident care.

The drawbacks of a large nursing home can be related to size as well. A large staff is simply harder to manage carefully than a smaller one. Unscrupulous staff members may be more likely to slip through the cracks and "get away" with things such as drug use or insufficient patient care because no one is watching all the time. The care provided in a large home is likely to be less personal than that provided in a smaller home because the staff may rotate more frequently. Be sure to ask whether your parent will be cared for by the same aides on a regular basis, or whether the aides rotate from day to day.

The ratio of staff to residents may be better in a large nursing home than in a small- or medium-sized one, but overall the level of staff education and experience may be lower. A 400-bed nursing home with one head nurse who oversees hundreds of aides may or may not compare favorably to a 120-bed nursing home with one head nurse who oversees only dozens of aides. Find out how many staff members attend to each resident and what level of experience and education these staff members have.

Who Owns the Nursing Home?

Some nursing homes are owned by private individuals or corporations and are operated for profit. Others are run by nonprofit organizations such as churches or charities. There are advantages and disadvantages with each, but, in the end, *type* of ownership is not what matters most. You'll have to weigh each facility against your particular situation and preferences. Profit-driven homes must offer a reasonably high-quality product or they quickly go out of business. Nonprofit homes are not bound by the need to return a profit, but they do have to at least break even to stay viable. Sometimes that break-even point can be reduced with the help of outside donors, but resources are often scarce and tightly controlled in both nonprofit and for-profit institutions.

Regardless of whether the home you are considering is privately owned or run by a nonprofit organization, you'll need to know the cultural underpinnings of the home and the level of flexibility and tolerance it exhibits. A home that caters to elderly Catholics may not be the right place for an eighty-two-year-old Reform Jew, but then again it may work out just fine, depending on the home's individual culture. Some long-term-care facilities, especially in larger cities, cater to certain ethnicities. Institutions such as these will take the language, food, customs, and activity preferences of a particular culture into account when developing their programs. A nursing home with a cultural specialization may be particularly beneficial for an elderly immigrant suffering from senility or some form of dementia. Often older residents will lose their more recently acquired language and default to their native tongue. It can be helpful and more comforting for them to have staff and other residents around who can communicate with them in their preferred language.

More important than any cultural rhetoric in the brochures is a facility's day-to-day atmosphere. You will have to visit the home to get a feel for it. It may be beautiful and clean, but the staff may be dissatisfied and cold. It may be shabby and untidy, but the residents may be laughing and chatting and happy to be there. Make sure the culture of the nursing home suits your parent's personality, no matter who runs the facility.

Paying for the Nursing Home

Always ask for a complete list, in writing, of each home's fees. Most facilities will list a daily rate. As of this writing, the daily rate averages somewhere between one hundred and two hundred dollars per day, depending upon the type of services offered and where the facility is located. Caveat emptor: Be sure to ask exactly what services are included in the daily rate.

Some nursing homes increase their daily rate depending on the type of care the resident requires. For example, the daily rate may be an affordable and competitive one hundred dollars at a beautiful nursing home, but you may discover it will cost quite a bit more if your parent needs help with meals or incontinence or medication. If your parent doesn't need that help now, he or she may very well need it in the near future. Some nursing homes quote a set price that includes all services, whether your parent needs them or not. Find out which is the case at each facility you are considering, and then crunch the numbers to learn how much each one is really going to cost you.

If you are planning to rely on your mother's or father's long-term-care insurance policy to pay the bills, be sure to read the fine print carefully. Many policies have a lifetime cap that limits how much they will pay in total, and they may only cover a short stay in a nursing home. While it is outside the scope of this book to explain all the various ways you can pay for a nursing home stay, many wonderful resources are available to help you figure this out. One explanation that is especially clear and easy to understand is available on the website MyZiva.net. (See Resources, located in the back of the book, for this listing and others that describe various funding options.)

Facilities and Services

All nursing homes may look different and offer different services, but some things are common to each. In this section we explain how to evaluate nursing homes based on the following criteria:

* Residents' rooms

* Community facilities

* Activities

* Therapy

* Daily and nightly rhythms

* Meals

* Connections to the local community

* Dementia care

* Pet policy

RESIDENTS' ROOMS

Among the first things most people want to see when considering a nursing home are the residents' rooms. The most important thing to do when evaluating a room for your loved one is to set aside your own tastes. It doesn't matter whether you like wall-to-wall carpeting or a spacious closet. What matters is what your parent is accustomed to and what he or she will prefer.

Other key factors to consider about the room include

* size and location

* furnishings

* private or shared occupancy

Small or large? Facing north or south? One person may feel lost in a very large room, and another may feel trapped in a small room. If the facility offers group activities, having a small room may motivate your parent to get out and get involved in community life, while a large, comfortable room may encourage your parent to stay isolated in his or her room all day. A beautiful ocean view may be paradise for one resident, but it may be unbearable for another who has cataracts or another vision impairment that makes reflected light painful. Be sure to take all your parent's needs into consideration when choosing a room and the placement of that room.

Furnishings: The furniture in a nursing home must meet both the working needs of the staff and the aesthetic and comfort needs of the residents. Some rooms come furnished and others are only partially furnished, but most will come with a special bed. The beds in nursing homes are usually more attractive than those in a hospital, but they have all the same electrical functions. Beds must be adjustable so residents can get into and out of them comfortably and staff can work at a level appropriate for their height.

Many residents in nursing homes have problems with incontinence, which makes carpeting in the rooms inconvenient and unsanitary. Even if your parent is not incontinent, the person who lived in the room prior to him or her may have been, and there is only so much a good carpet cleaner can do.

The best nursing homes allow residents to decorate their rooms as they please. Photographs, framed prints, calendars, and grandchildren's drawings should not be banned simply to keep the room uniform and tidy. The most important items in the room may end up being Dad's worn-out recliner and the ratty old blanket he always had over his legs when he napped in front of the television.

Private or shared occupancy: Those of us born during the baby boomer generation tend to prefer private rooms. We were usually raised with plenty of space and privacy and have come to regard having our own space as an important option, if not a downright necessity. But if the room we are considering is for our parent, we need to stop and think of what his or her life has been like. Did your parent grow up among siblings? If so, they probably shared a lively and noisy environment. Did your parent attend summer camp, sleep in a college dormitory, or bunk with others during military service? Many times people who think they would prefer a private room actually do much better over the long term in a shared situation. The sights and sounds produced by another person can be comforting. Having a roommate can give your loved one someone else to take care of and interact with; it can remind them of their youth, it can keep them from feeling isolated, and it can be of immense value if your parent needs help and is feeling too weak to press the call button.

If a resident is bed bound, a shared room is even more important. Bed-bound residents are consigned to staying in their room all day. If no one is there with them, they can develop extreme sensory deprivation. The worst punishment most prisons inflict is solitary confinement. Bed-bound nursing home residents in private rooms are not far removed from that awful situation.

COMMUNITY FACILITIES

Community facilities encompass all those amenities we grown children of nursing home residents love to see when we look at the brochures. We love to think of our parents living in a home with a nice garden, a living room, meeting rooms, fancy dining rooms, and maybe even a swimming pool. But what is more important than the facilities themselves are the activities that take place in them, and this is why we've included the next section.

ACTIVITIES

What kinds of activities are offered in the home you are considering, and what does your parent like to do? Will your parent be drawn to the type of eye-catching activities that are often used in public-relations literature to recruit new residents? Or is your parent more likely to participate in everyday, "real-life" types of activities? A good nursing home will offer both formal and informal activities. A youth concert or a wheelchair exercise class may be popular and well-attended, but a volunteer who quietly sits in the corner knitting may be just as interesting and appealing to your particular parent. Typical activities may include things like in-house discussion groups, walks around the neighborhood, attending cultural events and religious services, shopping excursions, trips to the zoo or bowling alley, and even the occasional vacation to a luxury resort that specializes in visitors with disabilities.

THERAPY

Nearly all nursing homes offer some form of therapy to residents who need it. The therapist may be either a member of the in-house staff or an outside provider who visits the home regularly. Nursing home staff is trained to know what kinds of therapies are suited to different medical conditions. Available therapies may include the following:

* Physical therapy

* Occupational therapy

* Music therapy

* Speech therapy

* Creative therapy

* Psychotherapy

The proper therapy will increase your loved one's quality of life by helping him or her maintain his or her current abilities, release tension, and feel as good as possible. In many cases it will even prolong your loved one's life.

THE RHYTHM OF THE DAY (AND NIGHT)

Each institution has its own structure and rhythms. One key to having a positive nursing home experience is to know how flexible or how rigid your particular facility is. Does your mother have to be in the breakfast room by 8:00 A.M. with no chance of getting breakfast if she arrives at 8:30? Perhaps the kitchen needs all the dishes back by exactly 9:00. If this is the case, the staff may be nervous about getting everyone fed quickly, which may not be the best atmosphere for your loved one if she likes to sleep late. Any organization that serves large numbers of people needs to have some systems in place. Find out which systems are rigidly enforced and which are flexible. Check on the consequences for breaking the rules, particularly if you think one or more may be difficult for your parent to follow.

Remember also to inquire about the nighttime schedule in the particular facility you are considering. In some institutions, nighttime begins at 5:00 P.M. and ends at 7:00 A.M.—and the facility expects residents to sleep during that entire time. This can be a very long night for some people. There may be organizational reasons to get residents bathed and into their pajamas by 5:00 P.M., but many places allow residents to continue with evening activities thereafter. Residents in these facilities can watch television, walk the halls, and even visit in-house "nightclubs" where they can share juice, tea, or soda with their fellow night owls. It is usually best if the home can allow residents to sleep based on their own internal clocks instead of forcing a schedule upon them.

MEALS

One hundred different residents will have one hundred different tastes in food. Even the best meal plan can't meet every person's needs and preferences. Take a look at the nursing home menu. Does it list appropriate generational favorites? You may prefer a seared ahi salad and cold pesto pasta, but your father may prefer a hearty beef stew or meatloaf and mashed potatoes. Many nursing home menus offer choices. That works well for most people, but it doesn't work so well for residents who suffer from some form of dementia. They will probably not remember what they ordered and will instead want something just like the person sitting next to or across the table from them.

All nursing homes should be able to respond to the special dietary needs associated with certain health conditions. Low-salt, sugar-free, vegetarian, and low-cholesterol meal alternatives should be readily available. If it is a small facility that promises "home-cooked" meals, take a special look at the kitchen. Institutional meal preparation is a very specialized business. The environment must be hygienic, and obvious cleanliness precautions must be in place. Food must be kept at the right temperature and properly wrapped. Ask who does the grocery shopping in a small facility, as that task alone can take a staff member off the floor for several hours each day.

If your parent requires liquid nutrition through a feeding tube, find out who pays for it and whether you'll get a reduction in normal meal costs.

CONNECTIONS TO THE LOCAL COMMUNITY

From time to time, various people and groups from the outside community will visit the nursing home. They may include individual volunteers or groups from a charity, church, or school. These community connections are very important for three reasons:

They bring life into the facility. Children singing, volunteers visiting, and clergy members praying all allow the older people to be stimulated in ways that aren't available to them otherwise.

They return to the community with increased awareness. People who have visited a nursing home have a better idea of what they are like. What was once only an idea for them now has a face.

Volunteers often walk out of the nursing home with a warm feeling that improves their overall image of nursing homes in general.

They offer an informal form of oversight and control. When large numbers of people see what goes on inside a nursing home, it is more difficult for the facility to hide anything it may be doing wrong. When community groups come through, they witness the daily events in the home. When nursing students return to school, they report on what they have seen and done in the facility. Selecting a nursing home that receives lots of visitors and has lots of activities going on that are linked to the outside community is one way to ensure that it harbors few secrets.

DEMENTIA CARE

Dementia is a complicated subject that we can't treat sufficiently here. The most well known form of dementia and memory impairment is Alzheimer's disease, but there are others, and their symptoms often appear very similar those of Alzheimer's. All forms of dementia may eventually result in complete disorientation in terms of time, location, people, and processes.

It is worth noting that some nursing homes are unsuitable for people who suffer from dementia. Too much traffic may cause confusion for a dementia patient. A home situated far out in the country may be scenic, but if people can get lost in the wilds, it may be dangerous as well. The staff may not be trained to work with dementia patients, or dementia care may not fit into the philosophy of the institution. Even if they call themselves nursing homes, some facilities prefer to limit the amount of actual nursing they do by accepting only residents who are willing and able to happily play chess or quietly read the *New York Times*. Finally, beware of the facility that accepts dementia patients but doesn't know how to properly work with, care for, or handle them. Some such facilities can be overly liberal in their use of restraints or sedatives.

Nursing homes that accept dementia patients usually handle them in one of two ways: They either segregate them into a separate "dementia-safe" environment or integrate them with the non-dementia patients. The advantages of segregation are that the residents can be attended to in a quiet, nonconfusing atmosphere. Also, some attempts are made at training the residents, who are accepted and respected even if they tell the same story a hundred times a day. Finally, the residents can talk to each other and make contact with new friends, and they won't disturb the more mentally sound residents, who live in another part of the facility. The disadvantage of a segregated environment is that an unpleasant social hierarchy often forms between those who are more and those who are less demented.

Integrated facilities treat dementia patients as normally as possible. The residents are a part of the mainstream environment and are not stigmatized by being "put away" in a special ward or unit. Integration can be easier or more difficult for patients depending on their level of dementia and the attitudes of the staff and other residents toward their condition.

There are pros and cons to each form of residence. Regardless of the level of segregation, dementia patients should not be seen as a burden but rather as a unique challenge—just like every other resident.

PETS

Check the pet policy at your target nursing home before making any promises to your parent regarding animals. If your elderly parent can still care for his or her small pet and if the facility allows animals, it may be best to encourage your parent to keep his or her animal companion. If your mother or father can no longer care for a pet, perhaps you can pay a neighborhood youth to visit your parent's room and care for the pet. If the facility's policy states that pets must be confined to the resident's room and your parent has a cat, be sure to determine whether the animal will be happy living in such a confined space.

By the way, your parent's dog is only ready for nursing home life if it enjoys constant admiration from large numbers of people. There will always be someone wanting to pet and adore a resident dog, which may be a problem if the dog feels defensive about its owner. If a dog barks when the night aide enters the room or bites when a staff member tries to bathe your loved one, you will be asked to remove it from the facility.

Some institutions have community pets that live in the building and are shared by all the residents. Others have a visiting policy for pets, to allow family members and friends to bring their animal companions to visit the residents. These scenarios allow every resident who is interested in the animals an opportunity to see and touch them regularly.

The Nursing Home Staff

When you visit potential nursing homes, be sure to inquire about the qualifications of the staff. Nursing homes in the United States are required to display their staffing schedule prominently, and figures are available for each category of nursing care indicating average personnel hours per resident, but the numbers do not tell the whole story. While staff-to-resident ratios are important, the quality of care each staff member provides is far more important. Are the staff members warm, relaxed, friendly, experienced, and satisfied with their jobs? Or are they tense, distant, and seemingly dissatisfied with the way they are being supervised? You can be sure those feelings—whatever they are—will be translated to your mother's or father's care.

A *special word about the ethnic background of the staff*: Discussions of ethnicity must be handled with extreme care and sensitivity to all concerned. There are really only a few simple ethnicity-related matters to be aware of when choosing a nursing home for your parent or other loved one. If you notice that the staff's ethnic appearance differs from that of your parent, it may make you feel uncomfortable at first. Fortunately, the ethnicity of a nursing home aide has nothing whatsoever to do with how well he or she can provide care to your loved one. Warm, loving, and skilled people come in all shapes, colors, and sizes, and it is a caring attitude that is most important in any nursing home. In fact, many cultures have a history of treating their elders respectfully, and this kind of upbringing can translate into wonderful work as a nursing home staff member.

One thing staff members and family members should keep in mind is that nursing home residents should never be made to feel excluded by virtue of the language spoken around them. The nursing home is their home, and it is exclusionary to speak a language that the residents cannot understand. The primary language used by the staff will depend on the culture, philosophy, and location of the nursing home, but whenever possible it should match the language that your loved one speaks most fluently. If your mother is a native English speaker and is being well cared for by warm and loving people who tend to speak another language to each other in front of her, ask politely whether they would mind using English when she is in the room. When choosing a nursing home, listen carefully to the language used by the staff when they communicate to each other within earshot of the residents.

Your First Visit

When you make your first visit to a nursing home, take along the Facility Checklist (below). Arrive at least fifteen or thirty minutes earlier than your appointment time so you can stroll around the corridors and get a feeling for the place. Do the residents seem comfortable? Are they just being themselves? It is normal for some nursing home residents to be depressed or even angry, just as it is normal for others to be happy and relaxed. A few may be napping in their chairs, but not everybody should be dozing at the same time. If nearly all the residents in the common area are napping at the same time, the facility may have a practice of overmedicating them, or they may simply be bored and not have enough interesting and stimulating activities available.

Look for a small group of residents collected in the lobby. In most nursing homes, there will be at least a few residents who don't want to take part in the traditional peer-group activities.

They may feel they are not as "old" or as sick as the other residents. These residents can actually represent an important control group for the facility. They are very aware of their fellow residents and will often report any unsafe behaviors or wandering residents who may try to leave the building. If no residents are loitering in the home's public areas, the institution's policy may be to restrict them from using those areas.

Notice how the staff reacts to your presence. Do they greet you or show no interest whatsoever? Do they make energetic eye contact and display a polite professionalism? Or do they seem overburdened, exhausted, or withdrawn? Remember that some cultural and ethnic systems teach people, especially women, that making eye contact is inappropriate, but it is still considered polite to acknowledge and greet others.

During your appointment with the admissions officer you will learn more about the institution's overall philosophy and admissions requirements, and you will be given a tour of the facilities. While on the tour take special note of the items mentioned on the following checklist.

Facility Checklist

This checklist has been adapted with generous permission from the website MyZiva.net (see Resources). We recommend that you take this list with you when you visit each nursing home, to help you evaluate it.

Tour the facility: Visit the facility you are interested in more than once and at different times of day. Observe staffing on evenings and weekends; this can reveal a lot about how the facility is staffed.

Services: Does the facility meet your needs? It's okay to observe group rehabilitation services, but ask first. Is sufficient attention given to each resident?

Fees: Request a written description of fees and all supplementary or optional charges.

Odor: Walk around the entire facility. Is there an odor anywhere? Ask about it.

Noise: What is the noise level? Are staff members calling out to each other down the hall?

Cleanliness: Is the facility clean? Are the floors free of spills? Are the staff wearing clean uniforms, etc.?

Lighting: Are the hallways well lit? How well are the residents' rooms and common areas lit?

Mealtime: Observe mealtime. Do the residents appear happy with the meals they are served? Look at the menu. Are the residents offered choices? Do you notice any residents having difficulty using a fork, spoon, or cup? Is someone available to help them? Are posters within view showing how to help someone who's choking?

Temperature: Does the air feel too cold or too hot? Are air conditioners blowing directly on residents? Are you comfortable?

Staff interactions: Observe staff interacting with each other, with residents, and with families or visitors. Do staff members treat the residents respectfully?

Satisfaction: Do residents appear happy? How about the staff? Speak with visiting families. You can request to attend a resident council meeting.

Privacy: Is there a place where you can visit privately with your loved one? Are staff members discussing patient care within hearing distance of other residents and visitors? All staff should knock on a resident's door before entering his/her room.

Credentials: Is the facility Medicare/Medicaid certified? Is the most recent federal/state survey posted in the lobby or a common area? Does the facility have any deficiencies on record as a result of government inspections? If so, ask to see a plan of correction. Is the facility accredited by JCAHO (Joint Commission on Accreditation of Healthcare Organizations)?

Staffing: Ask about the ratios of nurses and certified nursing assistants per resident. This should be posted in a common area. Are the specialty units, such as dementia, short-term rehabilitation, or ventilator units, staffed differently?

Resident care: Are the residents well-groomed and appropriately dressed? Are they comfortably positioned?

Security: How does the facility protect residents from wandering outside? How easy was it for you to get into the facility? Were you asked for identification and the reason for your visit? Ask how residents' personal items are protected.

Safety: Are residents assisted when needed? Check for smoke detectors, fire alarms, and sprinkler systems. Ask if the facility has a procedure in place to screen for abuse and neglect.

Communication: What language is the staff speaking? Can they communicate with you and your loved one?

Mobility: Are hallways and rooms clear so residents can move around freely? Are there obstacles in the way such as linen, medication, and/or cleaning carts? These should all be placed on one side of the hallway.

Activities: Review the monthly activity calendar. Is there a variety? Can residents make a choice?

Postings: In addition to surveys, look for information on resident rights, the state ombudsperson, and the state department of health hotline number.

If you take into consideration all the factors we've discussed, the result will be that intangible quality we call atmosphere. A comfortable, inviting atmosphere in a nursing home is the most important thing you can look for because it will come as a result of the other factors being in order. If you walk into a nursing home and don't feel good about the atmosphere, head back out the door. You may not know exactly why you don't feel good about the place, but trust your intuition and keep looking. Nursing homes with warm, loving, inviting environments do exist. Keep looking and you'll find one.

Taking Your Parent with You when You Visit

If your parent is of sound mind and has sufficient physical strength, you may want to consider bringing him or her along when you visit nursing homes for the first time. Sometimes, when a parent is resisting the decision, taking them to three or four facilities and letting them have their say about which one they like best will help them retain a sense of control. Sometimes just seeing a facility can help your loved one feel more relaxed and confident about the overall decision. Be sure to limit the number of homes to choose from or you could be looking at nursing homes for years to come.

On the other hand, if your parent is not physically strong, visiting multiple nursing homes may be exhausting. Your parent may prefer that you make the first visit and then take him or her to only the one or two facilities you have found most satisfactory.

Waiting Lists

If the facility you like best is 100 percent occupied at the moment, you can ask to be put on the waiting list. This gives you a chance to sign up for a future opening in the facility, but you won't know when it will happen. No one can predict when a current resident will leave a facility. It could be in a week, or it could be in two years. Even if one of the residents is in the terminal stages of a disease, today's medical care is so advanced that the dying process can take months. If you are number ten or even twenty on the waiting list, don't despair. It is the nature of waiting lists to collapse when tested. Most of the people above you on the list may have gone elsewhere by the time they are actually offered a spot in the home, and you may be offered something the very next week.

If you have your heart set on a particular home and it is full, get your name on the waiting list and call at least once a month to reconfirm your interest. Regular contact will let the director know your interest is sincere, and after the first few people on the list turn down a placement he or she may jump right down to your name because it is certain that you will take the available spot. Nursing home administrators don't have a lot of time to recruit new residents. Being in the right place at the right time can make the difference, and calling regularly will help you be in that right place and time.

If your parent is on the waiting list for a shared room, be aware that you may not be offered the first place available when it is your turn. Other factors have to be considered, including the sex of the roommate in the available room, his or her health condition, and his or her personality type. If the only available bed is in a room shared with a severely demented or aggressive roommate, the staff may have to look farther down the list for someone more compatible. Waiting lists are also impacted by the level of care required by the resident to be admitted. Not all nursing homes are capable of caring for all conditions. For example, if the potential resident is in a coma, taking care of him or her will require a lot of physical effort and heavy lifting on the part of the staff. If the home happens to have three pregnant aides, it may very well be unable to accept a comatose resident.

In any case, don't feel bad if you hear "Sorry, but no" from a facility you were hoping would accept your parent. A well-reasoned no is far better than an unsuitable yes. When your mother's or father's safety and quality of life are at stake, don't urge, push, plead, or beg to be granted an exception. Keep looking. Trust that it is for the best. Get your parent into a place that feels comfortable and confident in accepting him or her, and everyone will be much better off in the long run.

Chapter *7*

Once You've Found a Facility You Like

After visiting several nursing homes, you've found just the right place for your parent. It feels right, it's affordable, and it has a room available now. You're almost ready. There are just a few more things to consider.

Talking It Over with Your Parent

If your parent has been part of the decision-making process, he or she will be interested and involved in what is happening. Communication can stay open, and you can keep your parent informed about developments. On the other hand, if you have not yet told your parent about the nursing home decision, the time to do so may now be at hand. First, though, you may want to reread Part I of this book. Once you've worked through the exercises on change and on expressing your feelings, you'll be more clear and confident about how to discuss the issue with your parent openly and honestly. We cannot guarantee that the conversation will be easy or painless, but it has to be done, and after reading this book you'll be as prepared as you can be. Remind yourself frequently that you're doing the best you can.

Sometimes it can be helpful to have a third party intervene on your behalf. If there is someone your parent trusts more than you at the moment, let that person do the talking. Let's return to Amy and Ruth, whom we last heard from in Chapter 5.

> Amy couldn't let her mother go home from the hospital, but Ruth was insisting on it, and the doctor considered her case merely a "hygienic problem." Fortunately, a nurse at the hospital had been through a similar problem with her own mother and offered to help. She told Ruth that it would be best for her to go to a rehabilitative nursing home for a short-term stay, just to get the sore on her leg attended to. She explained that the nursing home had special tools for handling "problem toenails" and special lotions for taking care of "dry skin." This explanation allowed Ruth to maintain her dignity and enter the home on the nurse's recommendation, with only a short-term stay in mind.

One cautionary note: Never tell your parent that the nursing home placement is only for a short time and that you'll take him or her home soon if you know this is not possible. Amy was hoping that Ruth would like living in the nursing home and would decide on her own to stay. But occasionally residents of nursing homes are waiting for their son or daughter to come and take them home— even though the staff knows it is never going to happen. These residents don't integrate themselves into the life of the community because they are perpetually planning to leave it behind. Eventually, when they realize they have been betrayed, they feel cheated and humiliated by their own family members.

If your parent is suffering from some form of dementia, there are different ways to let him or her know about the impending nursing home admission. The best strategy may be to take your loved one along on a visit to the facility. After meeting with your parent, the staff psychologist, team leader, or social worker can advise you how best to tell your parent about the imminent move.

If other people are involved in the nursing home decision, such as your spouse or siblings, make sure everyone is on the same page.

If you keep everyone informed about the process and how it is going, there will be fewer conflicts later on. Many nursing home residents have been troubled by the fact that some of their children support their having entered a nursing home while others view it as a horrible thing.

Preparing Clothing and Other Possessions

You'll probably receive a checklist from the nursing home about its requirements regarding clothing and other personal possessions your parent will need in the facility. Ask whether you should label your parent's clothing or whether the institution uses its own electronic labeling system to allow for scanning and sorting of the laundry. Of course, you can do both. Sometimes using name labels is helpful even in a facility that uses barcode labeling, because the barcodes can be read only by the scanning machine and not by the staff or the resident.

Remember to label your loved one's furniture as well, so it doesn't get mixed in with the institution's furniture. If your father has his favorite chair in his room, for example, but he can no longer walk, the staff may need to move the chair out of the room to accommodate his wheelchair. If your father's chair is not labeled, a staff member may assume it belongs to the facility and simply put it in the common room or allow another resident to use it.

Keeping Your Parent's House or Apartment

If your parent is feeling halfhearted about the nursing home decision or is resisting it altogether, you may want to consider an honest attempt to make the stay a short-term, rehabilitative one. If this is at all possible, be sure to keep your parent's apartment or house available for his or her return. Once your mother or father has experienced the ease of having someone else do their laundry and cook their meals, they may never want to return to their former home. At the same time, many residents like knowing their home is there for them. Some families keep their mother's or father's home "on hold" for their parent for several years, until the nursing home stay becomes more obviously a permanent one.

Moving In and Feeling at Home Are Two Different Things

When anyone moves into any new residence, getting settled in is more of a process than an event. It can take some time before you feel at home in your new dwelling. Getting settled into a nursing home is no exception. It usually takes from three to six weeks, or even longer, before a new resident begins to feel comfortable in his or her surroundings, and then it only happens if the resident feels as if life is worth living in his or her particular nursing home.

Every resident will adjust in his or her own time and own way, but certain patterns are consistent among all residents. New nursing home residents tend to fall into five different groups:

1. Hospital arrivals

2. Putting my best face forward

3. I'll go, but I won't like it

4. No way, no how!

5. Ready, willing, and able

HOSPITAL ARRIVALS

These new residents are usually suffering from a long-term illness. Most have been recently discharged from the hospital and cannot return to their own home. They usually feel very weak and may be semiconscious. When they arrive they usually adjust quickly, because life in a nursing home is often more comfortable and welcoming than life in a hospital. From the first day, the nursing home may represent an improvement over the hospital they've just left, so they accept it easily.

Of course, some of these residents are so weak they are not even aware of the move. They may adjust immediately to nursing home life, or they may experience a delayed and more gradual adjustment as their condition improves and they become stronger and more aware of their surroundings.

PUTTING MY BEST FACE FORWARD

Some new residents arrive putting their best face forward. They have been prepared for the move, they have agreed to it, and they are on their best behavior. They may compliment the staff, make positive remarks about the facilities and the food, and in general have a very easy time moving in. In Germany, this group is referred to as showing only their "chocolate" side, or sweeter side, at first.

Since they are human, they won't be able to be at their best forever. They may experience some kind of crisis around the second week after admission. They may suddenly become aware of all the imperfections, both real and imagined, of the nursing home. They may endure a period when nothing is good enough and nothing satisfies them. They may complain about everything and say they don't like it there anymore.

After swinging from one emotional extreme to the other, residents in this group begin to feel at home after a week or two of complaining. Eventually they settle into a state where they can be themselves, experiencing all the normal highs and lows they had before moving in. They may not end up loving everything about the nursing home, but they probably won't hate everything about it, either.

I'LL GO, BUT I WON'T LIKE IT!

Maybe your father has agreed to move into a nursing home because it is the most logical solution, but perhaps on an emotional level he doesn't really want to. Initially, he may appear withdrawn and even surly. He is there but he does not participate. He is observing and getting a feel for the community, but is not quite a part of it. He feels lost, and it seems as if the facility has nothing to offer him. He doesn't know how to feel at home there.

If this describes your parent, a good nursing home staff will regularly and subtly encourage him or her to try each of the community activities at least once. The aides will gently try to engage your loved one in different activities until he or she finds something he or she likes to do. Also, in a case like the one described above, the staff will accept those times when your father doesn't want to take part in an activity, but will keep encouraging him with a gentle and friendly manner.

Residents in this group usually take a good two or three weeks to come out of their shell after arriving at the nursing home. They will make friends more slowly and carefully than some of the other residents, but those friendships will often be more lasting and stable. Although you may never see your father on television praising his nursing home and saying it is the best place on earth, if after a few months you ask him whether he wants to leave, he will probably tell you, "No!"

NO WAY, NO HOW!

Residents in this group are often those who are forced to live in a nursing home, usually by their health condition or other circumstances, but who do not want to be there. They are often angry about the placement and may refuse to take part in anything at all for several weeks. If the staff keeps trying to engage them, they usually come around, but it can take some time.

> Our friend Charley had always been a very athletic and independent man who enjoyed being outdoors and taking part in physical activities. One day Charley had a stroke, and after some time in the hospital he found himself partially paralyzed and living in a nursing home. Charley was hostile and rude to the staff and the other residents. He did not want to be there. Most people didn't want to go near him. When Sharon, the physical therapist, came to his room, he would yell at her and insist that she leave immediately.

Fortunately for Charley, Sharon didn't give up on him. She came back day after day. And day after day Charley threw her out of his room. Sharon had been coming to Charley's room every day for nearly eight weeks before he finally let her stay. After that he began taking his physical therapy regularly. He now feels quite a bit more at home in his nursing home. He still does not like the idea of living a compromised existence, but he is slowly regaining some abilities that will allow him to experience life more fully.

The danger for residents in this group is that their hostility and anger may drive the staff away completely. After some time of being abused and rebuffed, staff members in some nursing homes may give up on an angry resident altogether. When this happens, these residents usually give up on themselves and prepare both mentally and physically for their lives to end.

READY, WILLING, AND ABLE

These are the residents who make themselves at home most quickly in a nursing home. They are ready both mentally and emotionally for the move to the nursing home. In many cases, they have some personal experience with the nursing home. Perhaps your mother volunteered there or visited friends there, or maybe she or someone she knew stayed there for a few weeks while recovering from hip-replacement surgery. Since she's already familiar with the place, she has a realistic view of what life is like there, and she knows what she's getting into. As you can probably guess, people who fit this description tend to make the smoothest and quickest transition to nursing home life.

Regardless of what type of resident your parent is on move-in day, know that there will be some good days and some not-so-good days ahead. Before you expect your parent to fully embrace the new experience, give him or her sufficient time to get adjusted, get familiar with the surroundings, get accustomed to the rhythm of life in the facility, and make some friends at his or her own pace and in his or her own way.

The First Day

As we pointed out in Chapter 2, all life changes are stressful, whether the change was eagerly anticipated, reluctantly agreed to, or a complete surprise. Moving into a nursing home can be even more stressful than starting a new job or going to a new school or moving to a new city. The new resident will have hopeful moments, anxious moments, and perhaps even some angry moments. Move-in day can be filled with so much sensory input and new information that it can be overwhelming to even the most energetic resident. There are so many new faces, sights, sounds, and smells. There are rules to learn and directions to follow. There may be long corridors to get lost in and dining rooms to find. Some facilities will assign a fellow resident to be a "buddy" to your parent and show him or her around for the first few days.

Do your best to keep your parent's first day in a nursing home as relaxed and casual as possible. Don't overwhelm your parent or yourself with too much nervous energy. Consider giving yourself a break sometime in the middle of the day. If you leave for a couple hours it may give your parent a chance to get his or her bearings. You can return in the evening or late afternoon, and you'll be more refreshed and relaxed yourself.

Be sure your parent knows where the daily schedules and facility guidelines are posted. Cafeteria menus, staff schedules, and activity calendars are usually posted in a central location. Make small but uplifting improvements to your parent's room each day for the first few days. Start by making sure there is an easily visible clock on the wall. Many residents lose their sense of time when they nap, and they may be unable to read their watch if they wake up in an agitated or disoriented state. The next day maybe you can hang pictures. On another day you can unpack your mother's favorite blanket, and maybe you can bring her favorite chair when you visit next.

The moving-in process always includes everyday activities like unpacking clothes and personal effects, but the atmosphere in the room will vary depending on your individual situation. At the end of the first day, you may leave feeling excited and hopeful, or beat up and exhausted. You may feel angry and tense, or worried and afraid it's not going to work out. There is no one right way to feel on move-in day—and that's true for both you and your parent. How things go will depends both on your relationship with your parent and also on how easily he or she adjusts to the new circumstances. Your feelings will also be affected by how many moving-in details you've handled that day, how much information you've been given, and how much is still left to do. No matter how you feel on the first day, you may feel exactly the opposite way in two weeks and then feel completely different two weeks after that. Let that be okay and you'll get through it all just fine. Reading Part III of this book can help. It provides a glimpse behind the scenes and offers lots of strategies for living well in a nursing home.

PART III

Making the Most of Life in a Nursing Home

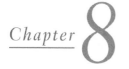

Chapter 8

A Day in the Life of a Nursing Home

Brenda, who was seventy-six when she arrived at Mountain View Nursing Home, had been a homemaker all her adult life. Her only child, a grown son, now lived in another state. She also had a history of depression.

After Brenda's husband died, a home-care service worker noticed her sluggish demeanor and the way her facial expressions rarely changed. He guessed that her condition was caused by her medication and suggested that she might be better off moving to a nursing home. Brenda reluctantly agreed.

After she had been a resident of Mountain View for three weeks, Brenda was evaluated by the facility's doctor. She told him the whole story of her life as he listened attentively. With tears in her eyes, she finished by saying, "And now, after all of it, I am here at Mountain View."

The doctor asked, "Does that make you feel sad?"

"Oh no!" Brenda replied, surprised at his conclusion. "I am very happy to be here. This place is so much better than living all alone at home."

One reason why nursing home life is often misunderstood and unappreciated is because most of us have never spent much time in one. We have little to base our opinions on outside of negative and sometimes horrific media portrayals. We may think of nursing homes as soulless warehouses for sick and dying people. We don't want to envision our future selves as sick or dying, so we may shudder at the thought of an entire facility filled with people who are ill and weak and needing care as they near the end of their lives. But nursing home life is just that: It is life. It is as lively and busy as life in any other home. In fact it is livelier and busier than life in most other homes. Just like "real life" on the outside, it can be upbeat and happy or it can be tense and stressful.

In this chapter we're going to take a look behind the doors at Mountain View Nursing Home. Mountain View is a fictionalized, composite facility, but the stories are all true. We've included them to help you feel more comfortable about "what goes on in those places."

What Around-the-Clock Care Looks Like

Care is provided twenty-four hours a day in a nursing home. (Here we're using "nursing home" in the narrow sense of the term—to mean the type of facility that provides ongoing medical care and observation.) During the morning, afternoon, evening, and night, your loved one is being attended to by trained staff members who are accustomed to helping people eat, wash, go to the bathroom, change clothing and diapers, and take medicine and therapies. If the facility is a medium-sized or large one, it will probably be divided into separate units of twenty to forty residents each. A team of staff members, including aides and nurses, will be assigned to each unit. The day and afternoon staff will probably be assigned at a ratio of one staff member for every seven to ten residents. The night shift will be smaller, with one staff member for every forty or so residents.

In this chapter you'll get a chance to see things from an insider's point of view. We'll spend a typical day with

    * Dolores, an aide at Mountain View Nursing Home

✳ Monica, Peter, and Sarah, three residents of Mountain View

✳ Harold, the facility's director

A Day in the Life of a Nursing Home Aide

When Dolores, age thirty-four, arrives at Mountain View at 6:30 A.M., it is still dark outside. She has been on her feet since 4:45. She got herself ready for the day, made lunch for her three-year-old twins, waited for the baby-sitter to arrive, and caught the 6:00 A.M. bus to work. When she gets to Mountain View, Dolores quickly changes her clothes and rushes to the morning team meeting in Unit Two, where she works. There she meets with her four coworkers, including her team leader, and members of the night shift, who are tired and ready to go home. The night shift fills in the morning shift in on what happened during the night shift. Rose, in room six, woke up, as usual, at 2:00 A.M. with her nightmares. Old Bill, in room eight, tried to go to the bathroom by himself and ended up falling again, but fortunately this time he wasn't injured. And Mr. Thomas, in room four, had a heart attack and was taken to the hospital. The day-shift team leader will call the hospital and check on him when the meeting is over.

Dolores scribbles a few notes and leaves the meeting. Now she will help six residents get out of bed, get washed, go to the bathroom, get dressed, and eat their breakfast. She begins with Mrs. Smith, in room two. She knocks at the door, enters the room, and opens the curtains. "Good morning, Mrs. Smith," she says. Dolores helps Mrs. Smith get out of bed and into the bathroom. While Mrs. Smith is on the toilet, Dolores prepares everything she needs to wash or shower the elderly lady. Then she bathes Mrs. Smith or helps her bathe herself. If Mrs. Smith is a stroke patient or is otherwise limited in movement, this is a good time for Dolores to work in some sensory stimulation. "Can you feel the warm water on your arm, Mrs. Smith?" Then Dolores assists Mrs. Smith in getting dressed. She makes Mrs. Smith's bed and takes her to the dining room for breakfast. There, another aide will assist Mrs. Smith with getting and eating her breakfast so Dolores can go off to wake up her next resident.

Dolores's goal is to help one resident get up and washed and dressed about every thirty minutes. Some take less time and some take much longer. Mrs. Johnson, in room twelve, is completely bedridden and can't go to the dining room. That means Dolores will have to get her breakfast for her and feed her in her bed. She'll need to sit with Mrs. Johnson while she eats, because she has a tendency to choke (aspirate) on her food. Dolores is always careful to cut everything on Mrs. Johnson's tray into tiny pieces before giving it to her.

Sometimes Dolores is able to work with two residents at the same time. Mr. Andersen and Mr. Wilson share room fourteen. While Mr. Wilson is in the bathroom, Mr. Andersen may begin slowly buttoning his shirt. Dolores can usually get both of them into the dining room at the same time, which allows her to spend extra time with Mrs. Johnson later on.

By 10:00, Dolores should have finished with all six of her residents, including making their beds. Dolores is lucky this morning that two of her residents, Sandra and Mrs. Smith, are rather mobile and only take about twelve minutes each to get up and get moving. Sandra asks to be taken to the bathroom every fifteen minutes or so because she forgets that she's already gone, but Dolores is used to this.

Since Sandra and Mrs. Smith can get ready quickly, Dolores has more time to spend with her two bedridden residents, Mrs. Johnson and Mr. Owens. They both require special care and attention in addition to receiving their breakfast in bed. Dolores needs help lifting and washing Mrs. Johnson and Mr. Owens because they cannot move on their own. Kadim, a nursing student who works as an intern at Mountain View, helps her out.

Dolores likes working at Mountain View. She gets to work with the same six residents nearly every day. She has gotten to know them well and genuinely enjoys their company. She has grown very attached to some of them. At the nursing home where Dolores used to work, she was responsible for caring for different residents every day. That facility treated the residents as "cases" and the aides as "resources." There, scheduling never took into account personal relationships between aides and residents, and only focused on how convenient things would be for the team leader. Dolores never felt close to her residents there. Mountain View is a much nicer place to work.

Every now and then Dolores is assigned to work in the dining room. When the residents come in, she greets them and brings them their food. Some of them, like Mrs. Walters, need help with every bite. Mrs. Walters simply does not remember how to eat. She happily comments on the beautiful colors on her plate, but has no idea what she's supposed to do with them. Dolores usually tries to seat her at the same table as Mr. Wilson, whom Dolores needs to keep a close eye on because he has a tendency to aspirate.

At 10:00 it's time for Dolores's half-hour morning break. At this time of the morning, many of the residents are still eating or in therapy sessions or watching television. Half of the staff will stay on the floor until the first group returns from break, and then they'll take their breaks. Mountain View has a staff break room where Dolores can have a cup of coffee. It feels good to sit down for a few minutes since she has been on her feet for more than five hours. She can make a quick call home to check on her kids. Of course, while Dolores is on break, some visiting family member (who most likely got out of bed at 8:00 A.M.) will probably walk in and see her drinking coffee or chatting on the phone. The visitor may say something nasty or rush off to complain to the director. Dolores is used to that, but it still hurts sometimes. She knows it's just part of the job.

At 10:30, Dolores finishes her break. Breakfast is over for the residents, and Mrs. Smith needs to be escorted to the hairdresser upstairs. When she gets back, Dolores begins sorting laundry and disposing of used diapers. Mountain View uses an outside laundry service, but the dirty clothes and linens must be sorted by the staff and taken to the pick-up area. She returns with the clean laundry from yesterday, which she distributes to the residents' rooms.

While Dolores is sorting laundry and helping residents to and from the bathroom, one of the team nurses takes care of the residents' medications. The nurse checks to see that everybody gets and takes his or her medicine. She may also give injections to the diabetics (and there are many diabetics). She checks blood pressure and blood sugar and calls the doctor if anything is amiss. If the facility is large it will have its own doctor on staff, but if the residents each have their own doctor, the nurse may have to know and communicate with twenty to forty different physicians on a frequent basis.

Several residents have wounds that need to be treated. Open sores on residents' legs are common since many older people have varicose veins or compromised blood circulation. Ideally, no one should have any bedsores, but people who check into the nursing home after having been inadequately cared for often arrive with some kind of pressure sores that need to be treated. Special mattresses and bedding materials are used to help avoid bedsores, but under certain conditions—if, for example, a resident is so weak that he or she can't move or heal—the sores simply can't be prevented. Sometimes older people develop "parchment skin," skin so thin that it breaks or tears easily. People with parchment skin get frequent bedsores and other types of wounds that need to be treated. Some residents, returning from the hospital after amputations or other surgeries, need their incision sites looked after. Some patients need to receive intravenous nutrition, hydration, or medicine. Their IVs must be checked, started, and stopped on a regular basis.

Between 11:00 and 12:00, Dolores helps each of her residents with their toileting needs. For some this means a trip to the bathroom, and for others it means a change of diapers and a washing. She also helps each resident with his or her exercises, prescribed by the physical therapist. She makes sure, with Kadim's help, to move all the bedridden residents, like Mrs. Johnson, into a new position every two hours. Residents in wheelchairs are lifted every two hours to shift their weight. At noon Dolores helps her more mobile residents to the dining room for lunch, and then goes back to feed Mrs. Johnson and Mr. Owens lunch in their beds. Throughout the day, Dolores frequently offers her residents water and juice. She encourages them to drink as much as possible to help them avoid dehydration.

At 1:00, Dolores sits down and begins writing into each resident's records everything that has taken place during the day. These reports are kept for the protection of the institution, in compliance with various laws, and to communicate with other staff members about each resident's care. Fortunately Dolores has been making notes on a small pad in her pocket all day, so all she has to do now is copy them into each resident's chart.

When the afternoon shift arrives, Dolores is ready for her day to end. Another team meeting is held to inform the newly arriving staff about all of the day's happenings. Most of the residents are napping so it's okay if no staff members are on the floor for a few minutes during the meeting. After each resident has been discussed individually, the meeting ends and the afternoon shift gets to work. Dolores is now free to go home to her children. She says goodbye to each of her residents and promises to see them again tomorrow.

A Day in the Life of Some Nursing Home Residents

Now let's take a look at the same day from the point of view of three residents of Mountain View Nursing Home.

MONICA

Monica is a seventy-eight-year-old widow with Parkinson's disease. It is 6:30 A.M. and she has been up since … well, she doesn't remember. She feels as if she has not slept all night. The night shift checked on her at 5:45 because she wanted to get up then. They told her it was too early. The aide gave her a drink of water, took her to the toilet, and escorted her back to bed. Now she is growing impatient. She wants to get up and get her breakfast and it seems to be taking an eternity. She pushes her call button at 6:45.

An aide tries to calm Monica, but she is getting more and more impatient. *Finally,* at 7:10 the nurse's aide comes to her room to help her get up, use the bathroom, and get dressed. Monica can walk very slowly, but she prefers to use a wheelchair because she's more mobile that way. She goes to the dining room and has breakfast. She loves watching the other people chatting with each other. At 8:30 she feels very tired and wants to take a nap in her room. She asks a nurse to take her to her room and help her into bed. At 10:00 she wants to get back up and go down to the lobby. She decides to attend an occupational therapy group event.

At lunchtime she doesn't want anything except a little bit of soup. After lunch, when her fellow residents are napping, she feels bored and wants something to happen. But all the nurses are sitting in the office and chatting. They are *not* working—she can see that very well because they are smiling and some of them are holding coffee. She's not paying this much money for the nurses to sit around and have fun. She gets irritated and starts knocking at the office door. She asks for help, saying she urgently needs to call her daughter. The nurses stop their talking. This is a daily routine for Monica. If they tell her they are having a meeting and ask her to wait a bit, she will go to the director and complain. Today they may help her or they may ask her to wait. Sometimes they give her the number, but she never actually phones her daughter.

After a few minutes, Monica goes into the common room to read the newspaper. She'll have a snack in the afternoon, take a nap at 3:00, and then take part in a group activity. She has two friends in the facility she generally sits with at dinner. The three ladies love to watch the older men, make comments about them, and complain about the food. Monica likes to go to bed right after dinner. By then she's exhausted. Of course, she wakes up at 10:00 P.M. and watches TV until 2:00 A.M. (Everybody is happy that her hearing is quite normal, because that means the television volume is not as loud as it could be.) She has another nap until 5:30 in the morning, when she wakes up and presses her call button.

Monica may enjoy complaining about certain aspects of her life in the nursing home, but she also enjoys the opportunities for communication, the activities she participates in, dining with her friends, and watching all the comings and goings. Monica's daughter, who lives in another state, feels guilty that her mother lives in a nursing home, but it's difficult to imagine Monica being happier in a home environment where there would most likely be far less sensory stimulation.

PETER

Peter, an eighty-two-year-old widower with diabetes, had already lost one foot and was having problems with the other when he arrived at Mountain View. Peter loves sleeping in and being the last one up in the morning. He really likes it when the pretty blonde nurse's aid comes into his room to wash him and help him get dressed. He doesn't usually smile at her but he loves that she's there and he tries to cooperate with her requests as much as possible. Peter also loves going to the dining room for breakfast. He really enjoys sitting at the table and looking at his meal before he begins eating it. What Peter can't stand, what he really *hates*, are those old ladies who always try to mother him. They fuss and tell him he should eat more. When Peter sees them coming, he hurries up with his meal to escape their attentions.

After breakfast, Peter sits in his special place down the corridor, where he's joined by Marcus, another elderly guy who can discuss the war with him. Peter and Marcus like to watch the nurses and comment to each other about them. Peter doesn't like the young ones with pierced noses or tattoos. He prefers the well-proportioned women in their early forties. Peter and Marcus love to sit and talk and people-watch and keep an eye on the window to see what cars are coming and going in the parking lot.

At lunchtime the aides always tell Peter not to eat so fast, but he loves his food and hates the old biddies who chat in the dining room. He just wants to get in and out of there so he can go take his afternoon nap. Peter has his own spot in the TV room, and everybody knows it. No other residents would try to park their wheelchairs there. Peter enjoys watching baseball in the evenings with the night-shift aides. This is his place. He loves being here and he has no desire to leave. He has never had a better time in his life.

SARAH

Sarah, eighty-seven, is a very sweet lady who loves people. She enjoys walking around the corridors of the nursing home and smiling at everyone she sees. If she sees a new person, she introduces herself very politely. "Hello, my name is Sarah. I'm eighty years old. I was born prematurely. I was a seven-month baby! Nobody thought I would survive, and now here I am. I'm eighty years old." Of course, since Sarah forgets, every person she meets is a "new" person, and they are new again in two minutes. Sarah introduces herself about a hundred times each day.

There are some bad people who don't smile back at Sarah. But she doesn't mind. She can always find a friendly person who smiles and listens to her introduce herself, and there is so much to do here. She likes to help the nice workers fold the towels and the napkins in exactly the right way. She takes her work very seriously and works hard to fold every corner just so. In Sarah's experience, if you know where to look, you can get very good food here. And there are always nice people to introduce yourself to as well.

A Day in the Life of a Nursing Home Director

When Harold, the director at Mountain View, arrives at work in the morning he is met with very different concerns from those that greet staff member Dolores or residents Monica, Peter, or Sarah. Before he even sits down he may find a message on his desk from the maintenance staff, telling him that the central heating or air conditioning has broken down again and that the repair bill this time will be unexpectedly high.

Harold spends his day making sure everything is running smoothly. At Mountain View, just as in all nursing homes, there is always food to purchase and prepare; there are staff to hire, train, and manage; and there is laundry to sort, garbage to dispose of, transportation to coordinate, and technology to maintain and update. There are also activities to plan, laws to comply with, family members to communicate with, new residents to recruit, public opinion to manage, and accounting to maintain. All this happens while residents are being provided with ongoing, daily care. So much work is involved in running a nursing home that roughly 25 percent of the staff are never even seen by residents or visiting family members.

Directing all the happenings at Mountain View is a considerable task for one person, but Harold loves his job and knows he's doing important work. The most challenging aspect, he says, is dealing with upset family members who talk to him or to staff members disrespectfully. We asked Harold if he had recommendations for family members who think that something about their parent's nursing home needs to improve. "We welcome everyone's input and help," he says. "Every suggestion has the potential to help make Mountain View a better place. We do appreciate people telling us when things aren't right. We just need them to understand that we're only human, and we have a lot of different needs to prioritize."

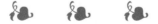

In any long-term situation, whether it be a family, a job, or a nursing home residency, it can be easy to start taking the good things for granted and to notice only the imperfections. This tendency can turn into a pattern of habitual dissatisfaction (discussed in Chapter 11), making it harder and harder to be content in general. So before you complain to the nursing home director, be sure you are seeing the good along with the imperfect—and take time to mention the good. This way you will know that your view of things is more realistic, and the director will see that your complaints are well reasoned. We offer tips in Chapters 10 and 11 for constructively dealing with conflicts in a nursing home and working with the nursing home staff. When everyone involved in a situation shows respect and concern for everyone else, the result can be a positive and satisfying nursing home experience for all parties involved.

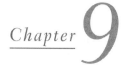

Chapter 9

Staying in Touch with Your Loved One Who Lives in a Nursing Home

"I'll never forget the first day when I left the nursing home and the door closed behind me," says our friend Diane. "I felt awful. It was like I had just put my mother away forever—like she would never be a part of the real world again."

If you feel like Diane, it's time for a paradigm shift—and that's what we're going to provide in this chapter. We understand that it sometimes seems as if a separate world exists behind the nursing home doors, but don't be daunted by those inanimate panels of wood, stone, or glass. You didn't lose your mother; you didn't "put away" your parent. Realize instead that you have hired a lot of skill, a lot of caring, a lot of knowledge, and a lot of specialized equipment. In fact, you haven't lost anything at all; you have only gained many resources. Visualize yourself as empowered by your new support staff. It's up to you to make the most of them. We're going to tell you exactly how to do this.

There are a number of ways for you to stay in touch with your loved one in a nursing home. You can write letters, call, and possibly even send e-mail, provided the facility has computers the residents can access. Of course you can visit, too. Visiting often seems to be the most challenging option for people, so that is what we have focused on here. This chapter addresses

* when to visit

* how often to visit

* how long to stay

* how many people to take

* what to do when you get there

It also includes a section describing a few special "staying-in-touch" activities, as well as a section on celebrating the holidays.

It is our sincere hope that when you have finished reading this chapter you will feel much better about nursing home visits. You will be more relaxed and in better spirits while visiting your loved one, and you will leave the nursing home feeling good about your visit, your relationship with your parent, and yourself.

When to Visit

Most nursing homes allow visits at any time, twenty-four hours a day. If you enjoy having a caregiving relationship with your parent or other loved one, you may want to visit when you can be of some assistance, such as during mealtimes.

> Joe visited his wife, Honey, in the nursing home every day. He arrived at lunchtime so he could help Honey with her meal, and he stayed until after dinner. He left to go home when Honey was ready to go to bed for the night. After many months in the nursing home, Honey died. A few months later, at Christmastime, Joe returned to the nursing home for a visit and asked if he could spend time there as a guest. He said he loved the atmosphere of the place. After that, Joe continued to visit regularly, chatting with the other residents and helping out where he could.

If you'd rather not take on the role of caregiver but would instead prefer to have a more leisure-oriented relationship, be sure to visit when your parent can spend some quality time with you. Avoid visiting during bathing times or therapy sessions, when your parent is otherwise occupied. You may feel out of place or uncomfortable just sitting there waiting for your parent.

Some nursing homes have official visiting hours, which can be advantageous to the residents. If visiting hours are predetermined, everyday care routines such as bathing and feeding are uninterrupted by visitors. Also, since visiting hours don't allow you to drop in when something else is scheduled, your parent won't have to, for example, feel conflicted over whether to attend a therapy session or spend time with you. But there can be drawbacks to a facility's having official visiting hours. It is often difficult for visitors to orchestrate their lives around the schedule of a nursing home. Residents who don't get any visits are very aware of *not* receiving guests during those two hours every day, and as a result may feel quite lonely. Also, be aware that in lower-quality institutions, a lot can be hidden from view if visiting hours are restricted. If you are a close family member of a resident who lives in a facility with restricted visiting hours, you can request permission to visit your loved one at times other than regular visiting hours. It may work well for you to do so occasionally.

If your parent does not need your constant attention, you may want to volunteer to help out with the other residents.

> Linda was an eighty-seven-year-old nursing home resident who could barely swallow her food. Everything on her plate had to be mashed, and it took her an hour and a half to eat even a scoop of potatoes. She could only eat with the help of visiting family members or volunteers.

Consider pitching in to assist a resident such as Linda. You can also help out by reading to a resident, putting together a jigsaw puzzle with someone, or just listening to residents tell their stories. Your parent may appreciate your being there without his or her having to entertain you directly.

If you want to help out as a volunteer, a good time to visit may be after dinner, when some residents always seem to need special attention. Maybe a resident had a nap before dinner and is now alert and wants something interesting to happen. That was the case with Davesh.

Davesh's son Raj was an attorney who always visited his father at 5:00 P.M., at the end of his working day. Davesh was never communicative when Raj was there. Davesh just sat and stared. Raj often felt uncomfortable and awkward during their visits.

A nurse noticed Raj's discomfort and told him that Davesh always had plenty of energy after dinner, and at that time he would usually go for a walk outside before going to bed. She suggested that Raj visit his father after the evening meal instead of before, when they could go walking together. Raj appreciated her suggestion and arranged to visit Davesh at 6:30 instead of at 5:00. Now the two men go walking every time Raj visits, and they both enjoy their time together much more.

How Often to Visit

"There's a nursing home right across the street from where I live," Lois explained to her elderly mother, Agnes. "Why don't you move in there, and then I can always come to see you?"

Lois meant well when she said those words, and her mother felt good hearing them, but the situation resulted in a serious conflict. Agnes took Lois at her word and moved into Lois's neighborhood nursing home, away from the one she had previously been living in and was accustomed to. But although Lois did her best to spend every free minute with her mother, Agnes was never happy. She spent their entire visit complaining about how long she had waited for Lois to get there. For her part, Lois was exhausted. She had no time to herself and continuously felt she was letting her mother down.

We can learn three things about nursing home visits from the story of Lois and Agnes:

1. Always be clear.

2. Underpromise and (if possible) overdeliver.

3. Be firm when your parent asks for more than you can promise.

ALWAYS BE CLEAR

It is important to clearly define how often you'll visit. Avoid vague terms and generalities. For Lois and Agnes, the word "always" meant one thing to Lois and a completely different thing to Agnes. When you commit to your next visit, make sure both you and your mother are in agreement about what you meant and what she heard.

UNDERPROMISE AND OVERDELIVER

When it comes to the frequency of nursing home visits, it is important not to overpromise. Don't say you'll be there every other day if you think you might be being overly optimistic. You just don't know what will come up, and your loved one may be devastated if you cannot honor your promise. As a general rule of thumb, we recommend committing to about half the number of visits you believe you are capable of making. If you think you can visit once a week, promise to visit once every two weeks. You can still drop in once a week, and your visit will be appreciated, but you won't be obligated to go there every single week if something comes up and you just can't make it.

Many people seem to believe that the more often they visit, the better. This may be true, but it depends upon your relationship with your parent, your parent's condition, and your lifestyle. Be sure to set a schedule that works easily and well for you.

> Susan, forty-eight, visited her mother Mabel, eight-four, every Wednesday. Wednesday had always been mother-daughter day for the two of them, and they each looked forward to it. Susan either would stay with Mabel at the nursing home, or would fold Mabel's wheelchair, put it into her car, and take her out shopping or on some other outing.

They lived in a small, rural town. One Wednesday, Rita, the nursing home director, was driving to work, and she saw Mabel sitting all alone in her wheelchair in the middle of a potato field, far away from the road. It was such a strange sight that Rita pulled her car off the road and ran to check on Mabel.

"Are you all right?" Rita asked.

"Oh, I'm just fine," Mabel replied, looking happily around the field.

"What are you doing out here all by yourself?" Rita asked.

"It's harvest time," Mabel said. "Susan is picking potatoes. I have a walkie-talkie right here." Mabel held up her radio and Rita laughed. She should have known that something as simple as a potato harvest would never get in the way of Mabel and Susan's special mother-daughter Wednesdays.

Look at the frequency of contact in your relationship with your parent before he or she entered a nursing home and try to visit with that same frequency. Did you visit your mother weekly? Monthly? The same will probably be just fine now that she is living in a nursing home.

There is one possible exception to the above guideline: In many cases it is best *not* to visit daily. Even if you've had a good relationship with your loved one and have spent lots of time with him or her, you don't need to show up at the nursing home every day. If you and your loved one have been together every day before the nursing home admission, consider visiting two or three times a week thereafter. Daily visitors can prevent a nursing home resident from becoming integrated into the life of the institution. Many old people whose well-meaning children show up every day like clockwork at 5:00 P.M. do not pay any attention to what is going on in the nursing home. They just sit and wait for 5:00, when their son or daughter will arrive. If you visit less frequently, your parent will be encouraged to get involved in the goings-on at the nursing home and in most cases will do so. She or he will make friends with the nursing home staff members, volunteers, and other residents. Additionally, if your parent expects you to visit daily and as a result hasn't assimilated into the institution, she or he will be devastated if you can't be there on any given day for any reason. If you have become your parent's entire social world, it will be much harder for him or her if you get sick, have a sick child, want to take a vacation, or have car trouble.

If you don't live near the facility, visiting once a month can be enough. Whatever your visiting habits, it is important that your parent be able trust in you. Never make a promise that you can't keep. This is more important now than ever.

BE FIRM WHEN YOUR PARENT ASKS FOR MORE THAN YOU CAN PROMISE

Never let your parent pressure you into making a promise you don't feel good about. Sometimes family members think they have to promise something because it's easy to do so in the moment, but the promise can come back to haunt them later and can damage their relationship with their loved one.

> Fred, age fifty-five, frequently visited his mother, Audrey, age seventy-nine, in her nursing home. At the end of each visit, Fred promised to come back soon. That was usually enough for Audrey, but one day she asked, "Will you come tomorrow?" Fred, a very busy bus driver, couldn't promise that, so he said, "I'll come by on Saturday."
>
> Audrey's eyes filled with tears. Fred felt so guilty that he said, "Okay, Mom, I'll try to come tomorrow." The next day, of course, Fred didn't manage to visit. And when he came the day after that, it was only for five minutes. Audrey, sad and angry, didn't appreciate his efforts to see her at all.

Fred needs to be firm and say, "Mom, I can promise you I'll be here on Saturday—that's for sure. I can try to come on another day, but I can't promise." That way, Audrey will know what to expect, and anything else Fred can manage will be appreciated as an extra. From now on, even if Fred sticks to his guns and only promises visits he can make, the relationship damage will have to be repaired, which may take several months. Audrey may continue to try to manipulate him into visiting her more often, and she may try to "punish" him with rude treatment when he does visit.

If you've got a parent like Audrey, don't give up, and don't let yourself be manipulated into promising anything you don't feel good about. If you remain consistent, clear, and firm in your promises, and if you keep coming back when you say you will, your relationship will eventually get better.

If your parent no longer recognizes you, it may be better to avoid visiting at all if what you expect is to be accepted as a son or daughter. If your mother is well enough to do so, she may have "adopted" some staff members as her "kids." She may literally feel as though she has a new family there, with no room for you. You may feel uncomfortable about the situation, but as long as your mother is happy, try to see it as a positive development for her *and* for you. You can leave the nursing home feeling good about having done the best you could for your parent. It is okay not to visit if doing so makes you feel bad, but stay in close communication with the staff. Call twice a week for updates. Sometimes people visit a nursing home to be near their parents, but while there they spend time with another resident who interacts more with them. You may find this solution to be more comfortable for you.

How Long to Visit

"It's so frustrating to visit my mother in the nursing home," said Frank, age forty-seven. "We have to drive for nearly two hours just to get there, and then my mom is exhausted after only a fifteen-minute visit. My wife is supportive, but I'm sure she'd rather be doing something else with her Sundays, and the kids absolutely hate the whole ordeal. They complain and whine for the entire trip. I love my mom, but, frankly, I'm not sure it's worth going at all."

Frustrations like Frank's are quite common among nursing home visitors. Family members often wonder how long their visit should be, especially when they have to travel some distance to get to the nursing home.

Depending on your particular situation, the best length for a nursing home visit can be five minutes or it can be five hours. Again, what is right for you will depend on your loved one's condition and on your relationship with him or her. A resident in a very weak condition may look forward the whole day to seeing you, and then five minutes after you arrive she may be so exhausted that you need to leave. When this happens, you may feel disappointed and useless. But even five minutes is worthwhile. For your loved one, it's just enough. It helps her feel secure and helps her realize she's not been forgotten. Nursing home residents have a different perception of time than the rest of us do, and five minutes can feel very satisfying to them.

> Fortunately for Frank and his family, their story has a happy ending. Frank took a week off from work, and he and his family visited the nursing home on Wednesday instead of on Sunday. They happened to meet Maureen, the facility's social worker, who spent some time listening to their frustrations. She offered Frank and his wife, Nellie, a valuable suggestion. She proposed that they learn about all the family-friendly and historic attractions in the area around the nursing home. Maureen gave Frank a brochure filled with advertisements for outings in the area.
>
> Now when Frank and his family get into their car on Sundays, their purpose is to have a fun family outing. They always stop in for a few minutes to visit Grandma on the way to or from their adventure, but the focus is no longer on the nursing home visit itself. Thanks to Maureen's advice and Frank's willingness to take it, Frank and Nellie and their family are much happier and more relaxed, and their Sundays are much more pleasant.

How Many People to Take when You Visit

How many people to take along on a nursing home visit depends both on the resident's condition and also on your family's expectations and traditions. Your father may love to have his room filled with guests, especially if he is from a large or extended family. On the other hand, if he's quite weak, more than one guest may tire him out quickly. Some people get nervous when there are more than two people in the room. They don't know where to focus their attention, and they get confused easily. These residents will most enjoy having only one visitor at a time.

Perhaps you find it difficult to decide whether to have the whole family go visit Grandma in the stiff family-reunion atmosphere you've always hated, or you just prefer to go by yourself. Chances are, if you make the kids go to the nursing home against their will, your whole family will be tense and unhappy when you arrive. After only a few trips you probably won't want to visit anymore, out of sheer frustration. Remember Frank and Nellie's situation. When they forced their children to visit Grandma, the whole family was unhappy. However, when they changed tack and took the family for Sunday afternoon outings that included visits to Grandma, everyone had a great time.

A special note on visiting with children: It's especially important not to force children to go to a nursing home. Some young people are very sensitive about being around sickness and weakness. If your child feels this way, it may be better for him or her not to visit for a while. Your child may be able to try again in a few months or weeks when he or she is a little older and has a better sense of what to expect. On the other hand, you also want to help your kids maintain a relationship with their elderly family members, even those who are sick. Do your best to be encouraging, loving, patient, and understanding, and their experience will more likely be a pleasant and uplifting one.

Many elderly people like to give their grandchildren a few coins when they visit. It makes the grandparents feel they are contributing something of value to their grandchild's life. This practice is fine, and you'll want to be sure your child thanks Grandma or Grandpa politely, but make equally sure your children don't come to view the nursing home simply as a place to get money. It will help if they have one or two other sources of coins as well. You may also want to bring along some coloring books, toys, and snacks so your children can play and entertain themselves while you visit with your parent.

About those residents who never seem to get any visitors: Family members often inquire about residents who never seem to have any visitors. The truth is there are some very lonely people in nursing homes who never get any visitors at all, but in most cases these people were "loners" before they came to live in the facility. Many people who live in the "real world" choose to isolate themselves from their communities, do not make friends, or have a lot of problems that cause other people not to want to be friends with them. When people like that change their residence to a nursing home, they don't suddenly change personalities. People who were isolated before will usually remain isolated in a nursing home. Likewise, people who were well-known and loved in their community generally get plenty of visits from friends, former neighbors, and family members.

What to Do During Your Visit

Once you've decided how often to visit your mother or father in the nursing home, you may wonder what to do when you're there. You may feel awkward and unsure about what to say or how your parent would like to spend time with you. This section offers some simple ideas about how to make nursing home visits more fulfilling and pleasant for both you and your loved one.

When people are old and weak, their nonphysical senses sometimes grow sharper. Your parent may sense if you are anxious or tense during your visit, or if you are bored or just "putting in your time" to fulfill an obligation. The most rewarding visits take place when both parties are feeling their best. They are relaxed and happy to see each other, and neither holds unspoken expectations about the other's behavior.

The first few times you walk into the nursing home, you'll be met with unfamiliar sights, sounds, and smells. Don't let that intimidate you or make you tense. You'll soon have a better sense of what to expect, and you'll become more comfortable with the place as a whole.

A visit with a resident can take place in a private area, such as the resident's room, where you'll be able to talk or just be together in a more intimate setting. Or it can take place in a public area of the facility, such as the common room or dining room, where you can be together with your parent and at the same time be a part of the larger nursing home community. A visit can even take place outside of the facility, say, at your home, during a walk around the block, or on a trip to the grocery store.

> For decades Jack Sr. had lived in a large house on top of a hill with a spectacular view. Now he lived in a nursing home that had no view at all. When Jack Jr. visited his father, he always felt uneasy in the nursing home but wasn't quite sure why. One day Jack Jr. suggested that he and his father go for a drive. Jack Jr. helped the his dad into his car and drove to the top of a nearby hill. Now, whenever Jack Jr. visits, the two men take a drive to the top of that hill. They sit together and enjoy the view while they talk and share a beer. Neither of them has ever mentioned the view itself; it just always feels right for them to be there.

Remind yourself that you're simply visiting your parent in his or her home. If it is possible to communicate verbally with your parent, talk about everyday life. Update your mother or father on all the latest family news. Let them know what's happening with their grandchildren and great-grandchildren. Be sure to update your loved one about any family acquaintances or friends who have died. This is very important to many older people. You may find that the most welcome topic of all is who is in worse condition than your parent. In short, just do what you've always done: Talk about daily life.

One easy way to fuel your conversations is to bring along a newsletter from your parent's church or another community group he or she belonged to. Or bring along the local paper from your parent's hometown. "I always try to bring something from my mother's previous life when I visit," says Noreen. "Last weekend, my husband and I attended a potluck supper at the church. I brought my mother a piece of Mrs. Dingle's famous blackberry cobbler. We had a lot of fun remembering Mrs. Dingle and eating that dessert together. My mother wondered who got to lick the baking spoon now that little Bobby Dingle is all grown up."

Of course you don't want to just talk all the time. At least half the time, maybe more, you should be listening. If your parent is fully engaged in his or her new home, there will be new topics for conversations. You'll hear about new friends, enemies, and all the dramas of nursing home life. One trap is very important to avoid, especially while you're in any public area of the nursing home: Don't encourage your mother or father to gossip or talk negatively about any staff member. Listen attentively, but don't encourage or participate in the conversation any more than necessary. If your mother or father is alleging an impropriety on the part of the nursing home staff, you may want to ask your parent calmly if there is something he or she wants you to do about it. In many cases your parent will say no. Perhaps your parent just wants to feel heard, or perhaps the complaint itself may have been exaggerated or even fabricated to gain your sympathy or attention. Sometimes people just need to complain about someone or something to get it off their chest. Once they've done so, they feel better and don't need to put any more energy into the situation. In these cases, after you've heard what your parent has to say, try to find another topic. If your parent has a legitimate complaint that you think needs to be addressed, see our suggestions in Chapter 10 for dealing with conflicts between residents and staff.

Be aware that by paying insufficient attention to less important news your parent wants to share, you may provoke a conversation about the nursing home's imperfections without realizing you're doing so. If you fail to listen when your mother tells you about Mrs. Brown's fourth-grade grandchild, but you perk up when she starts talking negatively about the staff, she'll catch on quickly that the way to get your attention is to criticize the nursing home. This may motivate her to embellish her tales. Most of us know when we are being paid close attention to, and nursing home residents are no exception. If your mother senses that you are eager to hear her negative stories, that's what you'll get.

If verbal communication with your parent is not possible, or even if it is, you probably can't simply chat for two straight hours. There usually just isn't that much to say. At home, maybe you'd watch TV or do something else. You can do something else at the nursing home, too. Bring your knitting or mending, leave the room with your parent and go to the dining room, walk in the garden, or watch other people. If your parent is able to do so, you can play chess or simple card games, such as Go Fish or Old Maid, or you can even put together a jigsaw puzzle. Board games such as checkers, Chinese checkers, and backgammon are often pleasant ways to pass the time.

Sometimes family members aren't accustomed to interacting with one another. They may love each other dearly but have always had a hard time communicating. In these cases, as much as possible, it's best to share the kinds of activities you enjoyed together in the past.

> After Henry had a stroke he was confined to a wheelchair in his nursing home. He'd never said very much, and he talked even less after his stroke. His son Ron visited often, but the younger man had never been much of a talker either. Both men seemed to feel awkward during their visits.
>
> Ron had an idea. He decided to take his father fishing, which was something they used to love doing together. Ron helped Henry into his pickup truck, folded his father's wheelchair and put it into the truck bed, and drove to a nearby pond. While Ron fished, Henry was able to enjoy the scenery and his son's quiet company. Neither man felt compelled to chat; they just enjoyed the time they were spending with each other. After that, Ron and Henry "went fishing" together often.

When verbal communication is impossible, usually your being there is valuable in and of itself. Just be in the same room, send thoughts of love, and hope that your loved one feels and is comforted by your presence. On the other hand, the opposite scenario can happen, too. Maybe the older person doesn't feel at all comfortable with you in the same room. Maybe he or she is afraid or somehow embarrassed. Be as sensitive as possible to your parent's reactions and facial expressions. Does he smile or frown when you walk in? Does she look at you or look away?

Sometimes your parent may indicate that he or she doesn't want to see you when you visit. If this is the case with your mother or father, you need to determine whether your parent is genuinely upset by your presence in a way that could make his or her condition worse, or whether your parent is merely trying to punish you or manipulate you into taking him or her home. The most effective form of punishment your parent may have available is to withhold love and approval. It can be painful if your mother or father responds angrily when you visit, but just know that such a reaction is probably a result of your parent's condition, and don't take it personally. If your parent clearly does not want you there, simply leave. You can try again in half an hour, but if he or she still refuses, try again on another day. You may want to reduce the frequency of your visits, but don't give up. Go for yourself, and stay open to the possibility of change. For help dealing with difficult emotions, review Chapter 5 of this book.

Let's revisit Amy and Ruth. Remember from Chapter 7 that Ruth was encouraged to enter a nursing home "for a short while" by a nurse at the hospital where Ruth was taken after she fell. Ruth agreed, but she remained hostile toward her daughter, Amy, even though she otherwise seemed to enjoy the nursing home.

"I really felt awful every time I visited my mom," Amy says. "No matter what I did, she would yell and tell me to go away and leave her alone. I almost stopped going. But I made an appointment with Marcus, the social worker at the nursing home. He told me that it might take some time, but not to give up. So I kept going back once a week. I would walk into my mother's room, and she would start yelling for me to leave. I dropped off a newspaper or magazine for her, checked to see if she needed any new socks or nightgowns, checked with the nurse to make sure Mom was okay, and left.

I'd be there for maybe ten minutes each time. I went back once a week for four months before she stopped yelling at me. One day she stood up and said, 'Let's take a walk,' and we did. Just like nothing had ever happened! I'm glad now that I kept going to visit."

If your parent is suffering from dementia, he or she may no longer recognize you at all. If your mother sees you as a stranger, you can show her photos, picture books, and other items to provide sensory stimulation. Give her different materials to touch. Consider building a board with different textures and objects attached. Then take her hand and gently touch it to each object several times. Do this with each hand. Ask the occupational therapist about exercises your mother can do, and help her with those. If she truly doesn't recognize you, consider another type of sensory stimulation that involves spending time with her neighbor while your mother sits nearby watching.

Be sure to offer your parent the stimulation of different sounds, too. Read aloud to your father from the newspaper. Don't worry if he doesn't seem to understand. Mental processes often happen inside a person's mind that we don't comprehend. Your father may seem to be asleep but may hear everything you say. You can read stories that you know your father enjoyed years ago, or bring CDs or cassette tapes of music that you know he loves. Make sure to bring his favorites, not yours. People often remember melodies and sometimes even the words to old songs long after they have forgotten nearly everything else. Sing Elvis or Bing Crosby or Frank Sinatra songs with your parents if those were their favorites. Give them different sound experiences each time you visit.

You can also bring some cologne for your mother to smell. Hand her a cushion or a stuffed animal to squeeze, depending on her preference. Or stimulate your father's sense of taste by bringing any food you know he loves. Bring him a gift of small chocolates, salami, or cheeses. Bring him a little extra to give away, maybe to an aide he especially likes. If the food you decide to bring is "forbidden" by your parent's diet (yet isn't likely to cause immediate harm, such as with a food allergy), be sure to tell the staff. A diabetic who eats a bit of chocolate cake, for example, may need an extra blood sugar test that day, or someone who retains fluids may need a bit more of their prescribed diuretic after eating some salty nuts.

Consider going out to a restaurant or to the park or to a shopping center, but avoid doing so during the weekend. Large crowds or too much sensory stimulation may exhaust or confuse your loved one. Get advice from the staff concerning the best and most appropriate outside trips for your particular parent. For some people, going to the supermarket could be quite an adventure, especially if they haven't been in several years. Others may like to go to a concert or a play if their hearing is good.

You Know More than You Think You Do

Trust your instincts, and utilize all your talents and resources when visiting your parent in the nursing home. Remember our aspiring gardener Beth? She eventually decided not to bring her mother, Gwen, into her home after Gwen's stroke, but instead found a good nursing home for her.

> At first Beth felt awful about her decision. Gwen seemed well cared for, but Beth had a hard time forgiving herself. When Beth later pursued her dreams of teaching gardening to schoolchildren and hosting a gardening show on television, she felt even worse. She felt guilty, as though she were living her own passions at the expense of her mother. When Beth visited Gwen, it was always with a sense of obligation. She felt terrible while she visited and worse when she left.
>
> Then one day, a nurse's aide asked Beth if she was the gardening lady on TV. When Beth said she was, the aide told Beth how much she loved the show. She asked if Beth could arrange some flowers in the dining room for the residents. Beth began to take notice of her mother's surroundings. She realized that a few plants and some well-placed flowers would greatly improve the atmosphere in both her mother's room and the common areas.

Beth enthusiastically took it upon herself to become the nursing home's "flower lady." Now when she visits Gwen, she does it with extreme joy and an armful of flowers. She knows she is making a positive difference in the lives of other people, and she feels good about it. "It took me nearly a year to stop punishing myself," Beth says. "Here I was, acting like it was the end of the world for my mother to go to a nursing home. I was making both of us miserable and I just didn't see it. I'm glad I finally woke up and stopped wallowing in my own pity party!"

Another resident, Hakim, had a daughter, Leila, who taught American history to high school students. During a unit she taught on oral history, her students visited the nursing home once a week for several months and collected stories from the older people to display on a timeline project at school. Both the nursing home residents and the students benefited greatly from the project.

Whatever you do during visits with your parent, do it in moderation. Avoid doing too much and avoid doing it all in one day. Get a sense of how much your parent or loved one can handle before he or she grows weary or overstimulated. For some people even sitting up in bed is a big change.

A visit to your parent in a nursing home should ideally be a time of joy and togetherness. Remember that what makes nursing home visits successful is not their length or frequency. It is their quality and regularity.

Special Activities for Staying in Touch

Here are a few ideas for keeping in contact with your loved one in a nursing home.

MAKE A VISITOR'S CALENDAR

Making a visitor's calendar for your parent can help him or her feel connected to you even when you are not there. It can also serve as a valuable communication tool between you and the staff members who care for your parent.

Making a visitor's calendar is easy. First, buy a wall calendar for your parent's room and some small stickers, such as colored dots. Choose a calendar with a theme and pictures that you know your loved one will enjoy, such as animals, art, nature, or other interesting images. Be sure to hang the calendar at the right height for your parent. If your father is in a wheelchair, you'll want to hang it lower on the wall than if he can stand up and walk.

Next, assign each regular visitor a color from the stickers, and make a "key" or sample chart. A visit from you could be represented on the calendar by a red dot. A visit from your spouse could be indicated by a green dot. Be sure that each child, grandchild, friend, and neighbor who visits has his or her own color. Place a dot of the appropriate color on each day you, or anyone else, visits. A staff member will likely be happy to use your dot system to indicate visits by others. Your parent will be able to refer to the dots and know that he or she has not been forgotten. If your mother cannot remember when anyone last visited her, the staff can console her by showing her the calendar and reminding her that you were there just last week (or last month, as the case may be).

MAKE A POSTCARD RACK

Most nursing home residents love to receive picture postcards. They are fun to read, fun to display, fun to share with others, and fun to look at again and again. The only question is how best to display them. If you put the postcards in a drawer, they may be forgotten or buried under the socks. If you tape them to the wall, your parent can see the lovely photos, but he or she can no longer read the message on the back. A postcard rack may be the perfect solution. Most nursing home residents will enjoy having one, and it is quite easy to build.

You'll need a thin board of the appropriate size for your parent's room, some nails, and some rubber bands. Pound the nails into the board, leaving the nail heads sticking out of the board by about ¼ inch. If you want to make the rack more decorative, you can paint the board and use attractive gold nails. Affix the board to the wall in your mother's room at a height she can easily reach.

When she receives a new picture postcard, which, of course, you will now send often, she or an aide can simply punch a small hole in one corner, thread a rubber band through the hole, and dangle the card from a nail on the board. The rack will add color to the room, and your mother will be able to flip the cards over or take them down to show them off to other residents.

PLAY AND RECORD A GAME OF "HOW WE DID IT"

Think of something you do today that your parents may have done very differently when they were your age. Ask them about it and record their answers with a video camera, a tape recorder, or simply in writing. Many members of today's older generation were raised during difficult circumstances and learned how to stretch a dollar in very creative ways. Ask your mother how she used to get new clothes, or build a fire, or entertain her younger brothers on a Saturday night. Ask your dad what his school lessons were like or what he did during church socials. Not only will a game of "How We Did It" bring you closer together as a family; you may also learn some very interesting things about your parent's early life.

How to Celebrate the Holidays when Your Parent Lives in a Nursing Home

Many nursing homes are centered around a particular cultural or religious tradition. If this is the case at your parent's facility, be sure to pay attention to the holidays from that tradition because as a resident your parent will be made highly aware of the particular elements of this tradition. The home will make these holidays an event, so you will need to acknowledge them, too. The staff of your loved one's nursing home should also know about the holidays of other religions represented among the residents. If it is a Christian nursing home and a Moslem resident lives there, the staff should know about Ramadan and how to properly celebrate and respect it.

The way you choose to celebrate the holidays will depend a great deal on how your family celebrated in the past. Whatever you decide to do, however, don't believe it when your father or mother says, "I don't want to celebrate." In most cases the older person doesn't want to deal with a lot of excitement, but nor does he or she want the holiday to be entirely neglected or want to be completely excluded from the family celebration. If your mother says, "Don't celebrate my birthday," send a card or a small gift anyway, or show up and make the day special somehow. Even residents with dementia will appreciate being treated with extra consideration on their special day.

HOME FOR THE HOLIDAYS?

You can invite your father or mother to your home for the holidays, but don't feel obligated to do so. A good nursing home will have a holiday event, which your parent will miss if he or she comes home with you. Some older people even grow anxious about missing activities at their home.

Your parent's ability to enjoy a day with your family also depends on his or her health condition. The travel and excitement may be too much for your mother or father. It can spoil your holiday if your parent begins coughing, choking, or vomiting, or is incontinent. If you're unsure how well it will work to bring your parent home, be sure the nursing home has a holiday event, and then visit your parent the next day. You'll be able to tell your mother or father everything that happened at home the day before and ask about the event at the nursing home.

GOOD GIFTS TO GIVE TO A NURSING HOME RESIDENT

Besides the suggestions listed below, ask the staff for other gift ideas for your parent.

* Enlarged old photographs of your loved one and family members. Scan and print them, and put them in a frame with a name label on the front. Old photos give the staff something to talk about with the resident. They also allow everyone to see how beautiful the resident was in her or his

younger days. Photos from a resident's past help the staff see the resident in a different light.

* Flowers (if your parent likes them)

* Plants (if he or she likes them and if there is someone to water them besides the staff)

* Lotions and hand creams in favorite scents

* A bottle of wine or special bubbly juice, if allowed

* Chocolates (enough to share)

* Homemade cookies

* A calendar with a theme your parent will enjoy

* Bed socks

* Slippers

* Robes

* Art supplies (crayons, paper, colored pencils)

* A personalized video of places where your loved one grew up. Include messages from special people. Watch the video together.

* Framed drawings by young grandchildren

* Large-piece jigsaw puzzles

* Large-print crosswords

* Large-print edition of *Reader's Digest* or another magazine you know your parent will enjoy

* For wheelchair-bound residents, a small mirror with a handle so they can see behind themselves (make sure the handle has a loop in it to allow them to hang the mirror from the chair)

* Food treats from your parent's ethnic background that he or she enjoyed during childhood: special sausages, liverwurst, sardines, etc.

* A reading light that can be attached to a book
* A book holder or tray for reading in bed or in a wheelchair
* A lap desk
* A magnifying glass
* A big, easy-to-see clock
* A DVD player with some of your parent's favorite old films or with a new DVD that you have made
* A CD player with their favorite music CDs
* A DVD showing Baby Emily's first steps or the first time she said "Grandma"
* A headphone radio (be sure to include time to spend teaching your loved one how to use it)
* Gift baskets of nonperishable items. These last awhile and look precious. Residents often like to show off their gift baskets to staff and other residents for weeks.

GIFTS *NOT* TO GIVE TO A NURSING HOME RESIDENT

* Wine to an alcoholic
* Chocolate to a diabetic
* Small items (which are easily lost)
* Stamps and stationery (unless you know from experience that your loved one enjoys writing letters and can keep track of the stamps)
* Knick-knacks for the shelf, unless they were made by the grandchildren (there generally isn't much space in a nursing home for display items)
* Precious things you wouldn't want your parent to lose
* Plants (if there is no one, other than staff members, to care for them)

∗ A basket of perishable foods, which may be too much for your parent to eat and will attract flies and bugs

Remember that a present is only a symbol of your love and appreciation. Sometimes it's better to give the wrong gift than no gift at all. Gifts don't have to be valuable to be heartfelt and uplifting. Even if you suspect that your parent will reject your gift, and even if his or her doing so will hurt, give it anyway, for yourself. That same person would probably hurt or reject you even if you gave them no present at all, so take the high road, keep trying, and know you did your best.

Chapter 10

Managing Common Conflicts in a Nursing Home

It would be nice if everyone matured into a pleasant, cheerful, up-beat little old lady or little old man. Unfortunately, the age-old question "can't we all just get along?" still applies, even when your parent moves into a nursing home. In fact, a nursing home presents entire new realms of potential conflict.

In this chapter we discuss some of the common conflicts that arise in nursing homes, and we offer suggestions to help you determine what to do (or not to do) about them. We address—

* conflicts between residents and family members

* conflicts between residents and other residents

* conflicts between residents and staff

* conflicts between family members and staff

* conflicts between family members other than the resident (i.e., siblings)

* conflicts within yourself

After reading this chapter you'll be better able to understand and deal with any conflict you or your parent may experience in the nursing home.

Conflicts Between Residents and Family Members

In this section we'll discuss both long-standing family conflicts and new conflicts that arise as a result of the nursing home placement.

OLD FAMILY CONFLICTS

The day your loved one enters a nursing home is not the first day of a new life for everyone. It won't cause old conflicts to disappear or be buried. In fact, long-standing family tensions may become even more pronounced because the stuff of everyday life has fallen away and all that's left is the conflict.

Patients with Alzheimer's disease or other forms of memory impairment provide a good illustration of how family tensions can linger. Even when these loved ones no longer recognize family members, they may retain emotional memories of past events.

> Laura, age eighty-three, had two children, Thomas and Carrie, both of whom were in their fifties. Her relationship with Thomas had always been rather peaceful, but her relationship with Carrie had been somewhat tense and troubled for a long time. The two women had always squabbled over everything, right down to the most minor issues. When Laura was living in a nursing home and suffering from memory impairment, despite the fact she no longer recognized either of her children, she enjoyed sitting peacefully with Thomas during his visits and still grew agitated and irritated whenever Carrie stopped by.

Even though old family tensions can arise when a parent moves into a nursing home, you can use this time as an opportunity to heal them. You now have a certain distance from old conflicts, and you are no longer burdened with your parent's everyday care. You can be more relaxed about his or her physical well-being. Do your best to see this time as a gift. You've been given one more chance to work on the past and heal the hurt places inside yourself. If you and your parent can move beyond painful feelings, you have the opportunity to begin forgiving both yourself and your parent for past mistakes. Nobody is perfect. We all have some forgiving to do. For many families, a parent's move to a nursing home is the wake-up call they need to stop taking each other for granted and start mending old hurts. If you and your parent are in the throes of a long-standing conflict, it may be worthwhile to hire a counselor or therapist to help you get through it. Reread Chapter 5 of this book, about dealing with your emotions.

Here is a practical suggestion you can start implementing immediately: Every time you visit your parent, before you enter the nursing home, take a moment to formulate a clear, positive intention for the visit. Imagine the visit going well and being enjoyable for both of you. Visualize pictures in your mind of you and your parent enjoying pleasant interactions. Hold that vision no matter what actually happens. By practicing a new way of seeing your relationship, you'll become more open to new possibilities, and ultimately you may even help your loved one see things in a different light.

NEW FAMILY CONFLICTS

Sometimes new conflicts arise between family members and residents as a result of the nursing home placement. Family members often find themselves in an emotional trap because a parent tries to make them feel guilty for placing him or her in a nursing home. As we pointed out earlier, if your parent has tried to control you in the past by withholding love or approval, or by otherwise manipulating your behavior, he or she will probably resort to the same tools now. One way to avoid taking the bait is to remind yourself on a regular basis why you made the nursing home decision in the first place. Sometimes older people who were unable to care for themselves at home feel so much better once their basic needs are being met in a nursing home that they find it easy to forget why they were moved there. They may accuse their children of placing them in the nursing home in error or for malicious reasons. If you allow yourself to forget all your sleepless nights or worried moments or nighttime phone calls, you may begin to doubt your own decision.

If your parent is doing his or her best to make you feel bad, write a note to remind yourself why you made the decision you did, and refer to that note before every visit.

Sometimes family members can experience jealousy once a parent enters a nursing home. It is normal for people to integrate into the community in which they live. Older people in nursing homes are no exception. Your parent may make new friends or grow very attached to the aides and nurses who help him or her with basic needs. If you feel yourself wanting more of your parent's attention than you are getting, it may affect your behavior toward your parent. You may find yourself complaining more or doing or saying unpleasant things just to get your parent's attention. If this is the case, it may be worth spending some time mentally reframing your relationship with your parent. Remind yourself that you are no longer the small child who needs your parent's constant attention to stay alive or develop self-esteem. Recognize that you, not your parent, are now responsible for your own mental and emotional well-being. Learn to obtain from other sources what you want from your parent. And be glad that your parent is developing a new circle of friends. Give yourself the opportunity to enjoy the time you have left with your parent. If you still have some feelings of insecurity, consider rereading the chapter in this book on handling your emotions or speaking with a trained therapist.

Conflicts Between Residents (or, the Battle of the Wheelchairs)

Anytime two people of any age and any condition are in a room together, the potential for conflict exists. Anytime a number of people who are all under stress, feel vulnerable, and aren't in terrific health live in close proximity to each other, a *vast* opportunity for conflict exists. If you've seen the movie *Grumpy Old Men*, starring Walter Matthau and Jack Lemon, just imagine all those little battles translated to a nursing home environment and you'll have a good idea of the kinds of potential conflicts residents can get into.

Whenever human beings live together, misunderstandings and rivalries can flourish. Add to this the fact that a nursing home is not a chosen community with a natural homogeneity. It is an artificial community where conflicts between residents are as normal and as frequent as conflicts between colleagues at work, neighbors, and family members at home. In fact, the frequency of conflicts may be even higher in a nursing home because of the artificial nature of the environment. Maybe your mother doesn't have anything in common with the woman who is sitting next to her. Maybe she doesn't feel the need to be diplomatic any longer. Even people who have been gracious and polite their whole lives can come to believe that they have nothing to lose by expressing their dissatisfactions in a nursing home.

Feeling poorly can also lead to crankiness. Many residents are not mobile; if they feel bad they can't even change their position. In normal life they could go for a walk, go for a hike, take a drive, or go to the gym to exercise. In a nursing home the residents have to stay in their wheelchairs or in their beds or in the common room. Residents of nursing homes must manage their aggressions without the opportunities for physical release that most nonresidents have.

Some resident conflicts are fairly common. Roommate incompatibility is a frequent complaint. Perhaps your loved one comes from a conservative, upper-class background and his or her roommate exhibits "improper" behaviors. Maybe the roommate is noisy and your parent has no peace. Occasionally two roommates have different natural rhythms—one wants to be up all night and the other wants to sleep. Generally, if a roommate conflict is seriously troubling, the nursing home will work with you to find another, more compatible person for your parent to live with. But before you run to the team leader with a request for a new roommate, be sure to read Chapter 11, on how to work with the nursing home staff, especially the section "Can't Get No Satisfaction: What to Do When There Is a Complaint." The good news is that most conflicts between people in nursing homes are not serious or life threatening. In fact, when viewed from a distance and from a neutral perspective, most nursing home conflicts can be seen as providing residents with the opportunity to experience a sense of superiority, relief from boredom, and a way to stay engaged with the world.

Sometimes a pair of residents may feud for years over seemingly silly things. You may think they hate each other, but if you look deeper you may see that they are simply keeping each other alive and engaged, like rival sports teams or verbal sparring partners. When one dies the other will grieve heavily and may also die very shortly thereafter.

If you see your parent or other residents embroiled in a dramatic exchange, don't do anything. In most cases it is simply real life, even if the blood pressure of both people rises. Don't take sides. You don't know the whole story. You can be diplomatic and discuss other topics, or be attentive and empathetic. Indicate that you can see how the situation seems very complicated. In one respect quarrels between elders are similar to quarrels between children on the playground. If you make the mistake of getting involved or taking sides, you may find yourself on the outside looking in when the two parties stop quarreling and make up. And although our parents are not like children, after all is said and done, life may indeed be a lot like a big playground.

Conflicts Between Residents and Staff

Interaction between residents and staff in a nursing home can provide fertile ground for conflict. In many cases it is simply a matter of each person having different paradigms. Nursing home residents often develop a different sense of time from those of us who live in the outside world. For example, your mother's aide may have told her, "I'll be back to get you in ten minutes," and then returned ten minutes later. To your mother, it may feel like an eternity has passed. She may complain that she "waited for hours and no one came." Or she may say, "It has been such a long time."

People with physical problems often become very body-centered. If your father is in a situation that he doesn't want to be in, such as sitting on the toilet and waiting for help to get off, it can feel like hours have passed even when it has only been a few minutes. Regardless of age, if a person is sitting in a wheelchair and something is pinching them, or they are sitting in bed and feel a pain, or they are walking along and suddenly get a cramp, even a short time can feel like an eternity.

Another reason for frequent conflicts between staff and residents is that some people may have become very self-centered after having lived alone for a long time before moving to the nursing home. Others may come into the nursing home from an environment that was totally centered around them.

> Georgiana, age seventy-eight, had dedicated her life to taking care of her tyrannical husband, Ed, age eighty. Ed was accustomed to Georgiana's waking him up each morning and handing him a steaming cup of coffee in bed. One morning, Georgiana suffered a heart attack in the kitchen and called for Ed. He refused to get out of bed to help her because he had not yet received his coffee. He lay in bed, furious, while she lay on the kitchen floor, helpless.
>
> Fortunately, the phone rang. It was Ed and Georgiana's daughter, Kathleen. She could tell immediately that something was wrong and called an ambulance to help her mother. It wasn't long before both Ed and Georgiana were living in a nursing home. You can imagine the kinds of conflicts Ed had with the staff, who were unable to wait on him in the manner to which he had become accustomed.
>
> As an interesting side note to this story, Georgiana met Ted in the nursing home and fell in love with him. She spent her days in the common room watching television with Ted, while Ed spent his days making trouble for the staff.

Nursing home staff members must split their time between different people with different needs. One resident may need help going to the toilet at the very same time that another resident wants her scarf adjusted. Both residents may insist that their need is urgent and both may insist that the aide help them immediately. If the aide gets a little impatient or flustered, one of the residents will undoubtedly complain that the staff is rude. If your mother complains that the aides are never there when she needs them or that they are being rude, try to help her understand that there may be someone in the facility who needs their help more urgently than she does.

Most of the conflicts that occur between residents and staff are very normal. They are the types of conflicts one might find in any service relationship, be it a grocery clerk helping shoppers or a waiter bringing food to customers. Conflicts such as these are usually based on different expectations. Since no one perfectly communicates about all their needs all of the time, and since many nursing home residents are impaired in their ability to grasp all of the dimensions of the larger situation at hand, some degree of conflict between residents and staff may be inevitable.

There are also times when the outer conflict is only a symptom of some underlying problem that may never fully come to light. Perhaps a certain staff member subconsciously reminds a resident of an old enemy or rival. Or maybe a particular resident is uncomfortable with the ethnicity of a staff member. Some residents simply aren't comfortable with needing someone to help them bathe and eat. They may act out against the aide to avoid feeling shame, vulnerability, or even caring attachment.

If you have ruled out the factors described in this section and are convinced that your parent has a legitimate reason to fear or dislike a particular staff member, read Chapter 11, "Working with the Nursing Home Staff," to figure out how to resolve the issue.

Conflicts Between Family Members and Staff

Some conflicts between family members and nursing home staff are caused by a family member's taking sides and forming opinions based on perceptions that are only part of the story.

One day, the director of a nursing home noticed the adult daughter of a resident looking very upset as she left the building. The director approached her and asked her what was wrong. "Up until now I was always satisfied with this institution," she replied, "but what I just saw has changed my whole attitude!"

Of course, the director wanted to know more. "I was sitting on the balcony with my mother," the woman continued. "There was a group of older people sitting with us enjoying the sunshine, and a nurse came up and began shouting at one of them for no reason at all. It was very rude. I was so upset I had to leave."

The whole story, of course, is that this particular old lady didn't hear well and refused to turn on her hearing aid. The nurse had to speak as loudly as possible to her. To an observer it seemed rude for the nurse to be yelling at the top of her voice, but it is simply impossible to speak tenderly to another person if you have to shout. Try it sometime. And always remember to get the whole story.

Annabel, eighty-four, had suffered a stroke. After only two days in the nursing home she began to react and smile, which warmed the hearts of the aides, nurses, and therapists. Everyone spent as much time as possible working with Annabel. Some aides even spent time with her during their break and after their shifts were over. Annabel was partially paralyzed and was unable to use the bathroom yet, so she wore adult diapers. Since she was on a diet of liquid nutrition, her bowel movements were very loose and runny. When loose stools are involved, diapers sometimes leak, and Annabel's clothes had to be changed several times each day. But the staff didn't mind. They genuinely wanted to help Annabel regain as much of her former self as she could. Gradually, Annabel began to communicate more and more with the staff. She continued to smile a lot. Everybody was thrilled at her progress.

Annabel's son Steven came to visit. He looked into his mother's drawer and saw only one folded nightgown. Without asking any questions, he threw a fit. "I was just in here four days ago with six new nightgowns for my mother," he yelled in a voice that carried down the hall. "Now there is only one left. That is mathematically impossible! What are you people doing around here?"

The aide on duty tried to calm Steven. She tried to explain that Annabel's nightgowns were in the laundry because her clothes had to be changed several times each day. But Steven refused to listen or to be calmed. He insisted on talking to the director immediately and threatened loudly to hire a lawyer and to take his mother out of "this dump."

Of course, Annabel was mortified by her son's behavior. She did not smile much that day. The staff members also felt awful. Nursing home staff members have to overcome frustrations like this every day. It is part of being a professional, but it is still hard.

Nursing home work is physically demanding and often stressful. The compassionate people who choose to care for our elders as a profession are often underpaid and usually receive little acknowledgement or respect. Don't make it any harder on anyone in a nursing home than you have to. If you have a need to find fault with other people's work, start with yourself and work to eliminate that need. If you want your parent to live well in his or her nursing home, be sure to get the whole story before you decide how to react—and then choose to react with reason.

As we mentioned earlier in the chapter, a sort of sibling rivalry can develop between staff members who care for a resident on a daily basis and the family members of that resident. The relationship between residents and staff members may become very close. Since there is no history between them, there is no baggage and there are no expectations. Some nursing home residents are even more relaxed in their relationship with a staff member than in their relationship with their children. Residents often psychologically "adopt" staff members. When this happens, the staff members can become like a stepfamily to the resident's "other" family—you!

Sometimes, very personal information is shared between resident and staff member.

Bernard was a well-known lawyer who was highly respected by the staff at his mother's nursing home. He was a local celebrity of sorts. One day, Bernard's mother, Rene, asked her aide, Irma, "Do you have children of your own?" Irma told her, "Yes, I have three. But I'm having a problem with my youngest. He isn't potty trained yet and he's nearly three and a half years old."

Rene replied, "Oh don't worry, I had the same problem with Bernie. He used to put the potty on his head instead of sitting on it!" The next afternoon when "Bernie" came to visit Rene, the whole staff giggled when they saw him. They were picturing the famous lawyer at age three, with his potty on his head. Bernard had no idea what they were giggling at and felt very uncomfortable.

For better or for worse, family members become like siblings to the staff. These relationships can develop the same problems many actual siblings have, such as petty jealousies and demands for more of a parent's attention. This is not an official part of the job for a nurse's aide; it happens at the emotional level as a natural consequence of the job. As we've already seen, you can't hide from emotions. They just are.

Your own emotions will matter in this situation, too. Some family members find themselves feeling jealous of a staff member and start looking for mistakes to blame on him or her. Of course, it is easy to find mistakes anywhere if one goes looking for them, and the situation in a nursing home is ripe for conflict. Sometimes hurt family members behave inappropriately by attacking a staff member about his or her hair, weight, or some other personal issue. Still others simply repress their bad feelings about visiting their parent.

One day you may notice that your mother smiles more at the staff members than at you. Perhaps she chats on and on about her aide's little daughter and doesn't even ask about her own grandchildren. If your mother expresses appreciation to the staff on a regular basis but does not even say "thank you" when you bring her a gift, or if your father flirts with the nurse's aide but no longer recognizes your mother, relax. The best thing that can possibly happen has happened. Your parent feels at home. You are now free to lead an unburdened life.

If you find yourself feeling a little jealous about your parent's new affection for the staff, take the time to find out what that little child inside of you still wants. Embrace the opportunity to develop independence. You are no longer dependent on Mom's or Dad's permission or approval for your sense of self. You are a free adult who can step out of the cycle of old relationship patterns and redefine yourself.

Of course, there are times when you may have a legitimate complaint about a nursing home staff member. If this is the case, or if you believe your parent's safety is at risk as a result of a particular staff member's behavior, read Chapter 11, "Working with the Nursing Home Staff," for ideas and advice about how to handle the situation.

Conflicts Between Family Members Other than the Resident

There is one type of conflict that can be very serious, can take a lot of time and energy from the staff, and can cause a lot of heartbreak and trouble for the resident: conflict between family members who live outside the nursing home.

Sometimes family members disagree about the nursing home decision itself. One adult child may say, "Mom, it is really for the best that you live here," while another child may visit the next day and say, "Mom, you know that if it were up to me, you wouldn't have to be here."

Intrafamily conflict—issues between grown children and/or their spouses—is nothing new to the nursing home environment. Generally such conflict consists of old issues being acted out on a new battleground and with new ammunition. Perhaps one sibling never felt she got enough of Dad's attention as a child and now tries to get it by sympathizing inappropriately about the nursing home decision. Perhaps another sibling who has had a tense relationship with Dad believes on some level that Dad is now most valuable because of his pension and wants to "bring him home to care for him."

Anne, seventy-nine, had always had very long hair that she wore in a bun. One day, Anne saw that her roommate, Cassie, had a new haircut and color, and Anne loved it. Cassie suggested that Anne try something new herself. Anne agreed and told the staff she wanted to make an appointment for a haircut and color. After checking with Anne's oldest daughter, Bonnie, the staff made the appointment.

Anne loved the results of her trip to the hairdresser. She happily showed off her new hairdo to the staff and her friends, who assured her they loved it as well. When Bonnie came to visit, she, too, admired Anne's cut. "It was a radical difference," Bonnie told us later, "but I could see that it made Mom happy, and that was great by me."

But Anne's happiness wasn't enough for her younger daughter, Brenda. When Brenda came to visit two weeks later, she was shocked by her mother's new appearance. She screamed loudly at the staff, "She cut off all her hair! How could you let my mother do such a thing?" Anne was in tears at Brenda's outburst. All the joy of her new haircut was gone.

This wasn't the first time that Brenda and Bonnie had disagreed. Sibling conflicts are as old as families themselves. The likelihood of a family having some kind of conflict based upon the nursing home decision increases with the number of children involved, their personalities and professions, and the family history.

Dealing with family issues takes a lot of time because they often involve several staff members. In Anne's case, the aides, the hairdresser, and the director all had to spend time discussing the matter. Morale suffered because everybody was happy with the new cut until Brenda injected her opinion. Anne was unhappy because her daughters were quarrelling and because Brenda wasn't honoring her decision. Everyone involved was frustrated, and the repercussions lasted for a while.

Since she didn't want to cause more conflict between her daughters, Anne simply stopped making decisions for herself. After the conflict, when the aides asked Anne if she wanted to go for a walk or participate in an event, she shrugged her shoulders. She was afraid she would make the wrong choice, so she simply stopped choosing altogether. Some time after that, Brenda accused her mother of being depressed and unable to decide anything for herself.

Sometimes family conflicts escalate to ridiculous levels. Often older people who are confused end up changing their last will and testament several times because a family member questions its contents. Some may put pressure on their parent to leave them something. A scheming son or daughter may say, "If you want to change your mind, do it now." The following week another child may say, "Did you know you changed your will?" The parent may say that he or she didn't change the will. Sometimes a pressured parent really is confused, sometimes he or she is just bored and trying to manipulate the family, and sometimes the parent is just trying to keep everyone happy.

If you find yourself enmeshed in family conflicts that negatively impact your parent who lives in a nursing home, get help. Many facilities have a social worker on staff who is familiar with these types of conflicts and knows how they affect the resident. Perhaps the social worker can refer you to helpful resources. Reread Chapter 5, on dealing with your emotions, and do the writing exercise provided there. Read the book *Peace in Everyday Relationships*, by Sheila Alson and Gayle B. Burnett, M.A. (see Suggested Reading List). And try some of the following strategies:

CHOOSE A PRIMARY DECISION MAKER

Just like proverbial chefs in the kitchen, sometimes having too many family members engaged in making decisions about an elderly parent can be more destructive than helpful. Even if your siblings have differing opinions about what to do with Mom or Dad, chances are only one or two are willing to step up and actually *do* anything about it. The others may just want to feel heard without taking on any real responsibility.

When multiple candidates are available to take charge of your loved one's care, it is best to try to agree on one person who will make the day-to-day decisions, be in contact with the nursing home, and be most responsive to your parent's changing needs. You might choose the person who lives closest to the nursing home, or perhaps the child with the warmest relationship with your parent. Some families instinctively allow most responsibilities to default to the oldest sibling, and others naturally assume gender-based roles. Regardless of which family member it is who steps up to the task of managing a parent's care, he or she will need to be sure that all the other family members feel like they are being heard. This does not necessarily mean changing strategies every time someone in the family has a complaint, but it does mean listening sympathetically and, if appropriate, explaining clearly and gently why things will be done a certain way.

Choosing a family decision maker works best when family relationships are relatively healthy. It also helps if the designated sibling is skilled at setting boundaries, communicating, and listening, and if the other siblings for the most part respect him or her. Family members who are not in the decision-making role need to realize that their wishes, while considered, may not be followed, and they must agree to make the occasional compromise. It is best to articulate these expectations and agreements very clearly up front and to intentionally choose the most appropriate family decision maker rather than letting things slide into a dynamic that gets complicated and messy ("Who made *you* the boss here?") and must be unraveled later.

In addition to electing a decision maker, some families may decide to choose a "peacemaker," if this role seems necessary and if one sibling has more skills in the emotional area than the others. Once these positions are filled, the other family members need to remember their own roles, and they must also agree not to talk negatively about the care decision directly to their parent. It may help if everyone concerned is made aware of the negative toll their bickering can take on their loved one.

KEEP INFORMATION OPEN TO EVERYONE

Even if there is one family decision maker, when more than one person is involved in the nursing home decision everyone has a right to have all the pertinent information available to them at all times. This does not mean the decision maker has to call everyone daily with every little detail, but it does mean that whoever is calling the shots must

* call them in the open (no covert activities)

* share the information fairly (no coffee klatches with one sibling without also updating the others)

* update everyone regularly and frequently (via a monthly e-mail, a news-filled form letter, or occasional phone calls)

If you find yourself making decisions about your parent's health or finances and wanting to keep them secret from other family members, you are caught in an unhealthy dynamic. Please get professional help in order to sort things out. As long as someone feels unheard or left out, there is huge potential for conflict that will very likely cause you far more stress than necessary and may even affect the quality of your loved one's experience.

"PASS THE BEAR": DEFUSE EXPLOSIVE CONVERSATIONS

Family communications can sometimes be fraught with so much tension that attempts at discussion prove worthless. Nothing gets decided, no one feels heard, and stress levels are elevated. If your family tends to have a hard time talking things out, try "passing the bear." Grab an old teddy bear, a pillow, or some revered family object (one family we know used their mother's old nut grinder), and set some rules. Let everyone know that he or she will have a chance to be heard, but everyone must first agree to the following guidelines:

1. The only person who is allowed to speak is the person currently holding the object.

2. The object will be passed willingly when the speaker is done. It is never to be grabbed or taken from anyone.

3. If your time (or patience) is limited, set a time limit (by using the timer on someone's watch or stove) for each speaker. The time limit may be five minutes or half an hour, but it must be the same number of minutes for everyone. If your time is not limited, each individual may take as long as he or she likes. If some family members abuse this privilege, simply revert to the timer system. No one has to speak for the entire allotted time—in fact, no one has to speak at all—but no one may speak longer than the allotted time.

4. The object will be passed in a logical order from one person to the next, until each person has had a full turn to discuss the subject while holding the object.

5. If a person chooses not to speak at all, he or she may pass the object to the next person, but his or her silence will be interpreted as consent. He or she may not "weigh in" later with a dissenting opinion. The same goes for participants who determine that the process is "silly" or a "waste of time" and want to leave. Anyone who wants to leave can leave, but his or her exit implies that he or she will defer to whatever solution the remaining group members come up with. There will be no opportunity to sway the decision later.

6. We advise you to begin this process with a question like "What do you hope to get from this session?" Then begin passing the object. Asking a question similar to this one helps to get everyone's expectations out in the open. You may then wish to continue with a series of questions—one at a time—such as, "What do you think we should do about Mom?" or, "What are your feelings about moving Mom to Mountain View Nursing Home?" and then pass the object around the room again. Or, after the initial question, you may just want to let the discussion stay open and flow where it may. In general, if your family members get along okay but are simply passionate and have differing

opinions, an unstructured conversation will work fine. If there are long-standing hostilities and tensions between people, the structured-question approach works well to help keep people on target.

7. After everyone has had an equal opportunity to speak and respond to the questions, *then* the floor is open and the object can be passed more randomly around the room to allow people to respond to each other. Use the following guidelines:

   – If you have something to say, wait until the person with the object is finished speaking, and then raise your hand to indicate you would like a turn. Chances are there will be other people who have something to say, too, so behave graciously if you are not chosen.

   – When someone is speaking, listen. It is not constructive to make comments or sounds, or to send other messages of disapproval. If you have something to say, jot it down so you will remember it when your turn comes, and then continue to listen. You may hear something you hadn't thought of before.

8. Occasionally, when a family member feels things aren't going his or her way, that person may try to sabotage the entire discussion. Since disrupting the process does not serve anyone, any participant may be removed from the process if more than half the people in the room feel he or she is not making a positive contribution. This is about family harmony and the quality of your loved one's life. All participants must agree to check their egos at the door. You may want to make copies these guidelines and have everyone sign a copy to indicate his or her consent.

   It sometimes helps to have a neutral moderator, such as a friend or even a hired mediator, present for these discussions. He or she can call the time and enforce the guidelines when appropriate. Just be sure the moderator is someone who is strong enough to do these things if the going gets tough and passions run high.

9. At the end of the session, pass the object one more time and have everyone answer the following question, "Are you satisfied with the outcome of this discussion, and if not, why?" If someone is unhappy, let that be okay. Just listen. Don't try to fix anything at this point. Remember that the object of the session is to help everyone feel heard and to allow everyone to air his or her opinions. It is not necessary to solve everyone's issues or make sure everyone is happy with the final decisions.

AND FINALLY...

If family tensions just won't let up, do yourself a favor and locate a good therapist to help you resolve any long-standing issues so that your parent can relax and feel more satisfied in the nursing home. If your family members won't go to counseling with you, go alone. Family dynamics have to start improving somewhere. Once you gain some clarity about what to do and how to interact in a healthier and more supportive way with your siblings, your family will be forced to treat you more respectfully. Some of them may even follow your good example and get into therapy for themselves.

Conflicts Within Yourself

Take time alone to make sure you are clear with yourself. Sometimes family members feel conflicted about their decision to place a parent in a nursing home. You may have a hundred good reasons to do so, yet on some level you may still feel guilty or uneasy about the decision. We hope this book has helped you feel better about your overall thought process and final decision. If you are still wondering whether you did the right thing, review the first few chapters and work through the exercises. Even if you have done the exercises before, you may be surprised to find that some of your responses have changed.

Take care to avoid the "happiness trap," which looks something like this: You have done all the research, worked through the decision-making process, chosen the nursing home, and moved your parent there. You have done the best you can do. Now you want your parent to be happy. But when you visit, your parent is angry one day, sad the next, dissatisfied with the dessert served during the lunch meal the following day, and complaining about the cold temperature on another day. You may get angry because you have tried everything. You may even fall into the cycle of trying to solve each day's complaints, but you feel worse and worse because you cannot make your parent happy.

If this sounds like you, you have fallen into the happiness trap. Your goal is unrealistic. You have done all you can, and now it is time to recognize that happiness is always the responsibility of each person for himself or herself. If your parent is satisfied at any level, let that be good enough. You've got your own happiness to be responsible for. Just as your parent isn't responsible for your happiness, neither are you responsible for your parent's.

Conflict is around us all the time. It is the most interesting ingredient in most of the stories we read and the movies we watch, and for some people it provides the spice of life. Remember that conflict is a normal part of life, both inside and outside of a nursing home. Not only is it unreasonable to strive for a conflict-free nursing home experience, but also often the best thing to do about a particular conflict is nothing at all.

Chapter 11

Working with the Nursing Home Staff

If your parent is in a long-term-care facility, sooner or later you are going to need something from someone who works there. In this chapter we explain how to work with the nursing home staff to get the best possible care for your loved one. If you haven't worked in a nursing home there are a few things you may be unaware of. Knowing those things and acting accordingly can make a difference between having staff members respond readily to your needs and having them seem unable or unwilling to comply with your requests.

Contrary to popular opinion, a nursing home can be a very satisfying place to work. Unlike in many jobs, if you are employed in a nursing home, every aspect of your personality is brought into your work. You can be yourself. You can communicate with others, build connections and relationships, and give and receive love, even from people who may on the surface seem rather grumpy, gruff, or downright unresponsive. Rather than being forced to stay in one area or to interact with the same one or two people for the whole day, you are free to move around and interact with many different folks. You can sing and dance and laugh and make jokes. You will be touched both physically and emotionally by the residents and your coworkers.

At the same time, if you work in a nursing home you can't hide your bad moods or your state of mind as easily as you might in some other professional environments. You may choose not to talk about your troubles, but they make themselves known in the way you speak, move, and touch the people you take care of. In most careers it's possible to hide your personal problems from the people you work with, but that's not the case if you're a nursing home aide. Try this exercise to prove it to yourself: Sit in a relaxed fashion in a chair with arms. Let your arms rest on the arms of the chair. Close your eyes and imagine yourself in a pleasant and relaxing location. Perhaps you're on a sunny beach, or fishing from a rowboat. Notice how relaxed your arm muscles are.

Now, without changing your position, think about a project you need to do. Maybe you are planning a garage sale or a wedding. Maybe you need to clean out the attic. As you think about your task, imagine all the things you need to get done. Are there invitations to send? Boxes to haul? Notice the muscles in your arms. They most likely feel a lot more tense than they did before you began thinking about the task ahead of you. If you were to touch someone when you were in this tense state, you would probably use a much firmer touch than you would if you were more relaxed. Nursing home aides regularly touch people in intimate and personal ways. Residents can sense if the aide is doing it with care and compassion and in a relaxed way, or in a distracted and tense way. The aide doesn't have to say a word. The residents just know.

We include this information to help give you a better understanding of what it's like to do the kind of job that reflects your every emotion. This awareness will improve your communication with (and, we hope, your respect for) the nursing home staff.

Communication in General

Open, honest communication is important for the well-being of any relationship, including the relationship between you and the staff members at your parent's nursing home. At its most basic, communication is the exchange of information. The information can be delivered or it can be received. In most conversations, information flows in both directions, but for the purposes of this discussion we'll describe each step separately.

WHEN YOU HAVE INFORMATION TO GIVE

Perhaps your mother has been complaining of cramps, or her wedding anniversary is coming up and you want to tell the staff. If you need to deliver some information to a staff member in a nursing home, always be sure he or she is ready to receive it. Do not say, "Oh, I've been meaning to tell you…" as the staff member passes you in the hallway with a tray of food in hand, or when he or she is in the middle of giving your mother a bath. Wait until the aide, nurse, or administrator can truly attend to what you are saying.

If you want to see changes made in some aspect of your parent's care, don't expect it to happen if you only offer a quick statement in passing. Write it down, and make sure the note gets to the appropriate staff member who can do something about your particular issue.

WHEN YOU NEED INFORMATION

If you want or need information about your loved one's care or situation, check first to see if you are entitled to receive that information. Depending on the circumstances, privacy laws in many states do not allow nursing home staff members to divulge information to residents' friends, neighbors, and sometimes even family members.

There are three elements to getting the information you need once you are confident you are allowed to receive it:

1. Find the right person.

2. Find the right time.

3. Find the right place.

Find the right person. Not all nursing home staff members are entitled to give out all types of information. Questions about medical diagnoses, patient condition, and drugs must be answered by a doctor or a licensed nurse. Even if an aide happens to know the answer to your medical question, he or she is not entitled to answer it. They simply do not have the adequate training to be sure of delivering the information properly and accurately. If you have a question regarding any medical prognosis, don't ask the aide. Ask the doctor or nurse.

If your question is related to the general care your parent is receiving, you can get that kind of information from staff members other than a doctor or nurse. Questions about how well your mother is eating, how much your father is sleeping, how her digestion is, or whether his missing blue shirt ever turned up can be answered by the aides assigned to your loved one's unit.

Find the right time. Many short questions have long answers. Be sensitive to the availability of the staff member you are speaking with. If he or she is very busy or otherwise occupied, ask if you can set aside time to talk later. Don't just insert yourself and your conversation between the staff members and their tasks. The residents' needs must come first in a nursing home. Your need for information may have to come a little later.

Find the right place. Be mindful of where you engage in personal conversations. Don't discuss your loved one's private issues in the corridor or living room, where others may overhear. And never discuss things in front of a dementia patient or comatose patient that you wouldn't discuss directly with him or her. You never know how much he or she can hear and understand, even if only on an emotional level. Sometimes coma patients awaken and report having been aware of events and conversations that took place in the room while they were comatose. Don't wonder aloud how long your parent will live, or bemoan the havoc his or her condition is inflicting on your schedule. Don't discuss the disposal of assets or argue with your siblings over your parent's care if your parent is within earshot. Always conduct yourself and your conversations as though the person being discussed could sit up and participate at any time.

One good strategy is to make a formal appointment once a month or so to speak with the team leader or unit leader about your loved one. The conversation can be in person or by telephone, and you can use the time to openly express any anxieties you may have about putting your parent in a nursing home. Letting the staff member know that you want to speak freely about your concerns is much better than silently projecting an attitude of suspicion and worry.

Showing Your Appreciation

Nursing home staff members are notoriously underappreciated in spite of the wonderful work that most of them do. We advise showing your appreciation as often as you reasonably can, but know that there are more and less appropriate ways to do so. If you want to express gratitude for the work of a nursing home staff member, be thoughtful when choosing your words. If you say, "Oh Agnes, I'm so glad you're helping my mother. I could *never* do this kind of work," you are actually being rather insulting. Agnes may feel humiliated to be told that the work she is doing is somehow inferior to the work that other people do.

You may be surprised to learn that most nursing home staff members like their jobs. They choose to work in the long-term-care industry because they are caring, loving people. Most of them would never trade their position in a nursing home to work in a loud, dirty factory, or stand at a cash register, or sit in a cubicle all day. For many aides, the worst part of working in a nursing home is not the job itself. The smells, the sick people, and the hostile family members are just a part of an otherwise rewarding routine. The worst part of the job is the social stigma attached to it by the media. Nursing home staff members return to work every day in spite of the ugly and incriminating way in which their work is often portrayed. Why do they do it? Because despite what you see on the television news, they know better.

Are all nursing home staff members open and honest and loving and caring and very nearly perfect? No, of course not. Each staff member has strengths and weaknesses. Some are much better than others at what they do; that's only natural. But nursing homes can't afford to keep the truly bad apples around for long. Most of the staff will be exactly right for such an important profession.

There are many ways to show your appreciation for a particularly helpful or pleasant nursing home staff member. Find out if any materials are needed for events, therapies, or other activities. Ask, "What can I donate?" or, "What do you need?" Sometimes a donation of simple items such as a few skeins of wool for knitting, paper for drawing, hardy plants, a bench for the garden, a new coffeemaker for the break room, or a few warm, wheelchair-sized blankets may be just the thing to make a staff member's working life easier and more pleasant. Or perhaps the staff would enjoy receiving a colorful gift basket filled with goodies that they can share among themselves.

Many nursing homes are frequently in need of new (or good-quality used) sofas and chairs. Since leather sofas are usually too cold for the residents, many facilities prefer the upholstered variety. But upholstered furniture is easily damaged by the leaky diapers worn by incontinent residents. Sofas are cleaned as often as possible, but eventually odors permanently set in, so they must frequently be replaced. If you want to show your appreciation for the care your parent is receiving, ask if the nursing home needs new furniture. Then keep this in mind the next time you redecorate or make a trip to your local thrift store.

TIPPING THE STAFF

Family members and residents often ask if they may tip a particular nursing home staff member. The answer depends on the tipping policy of the facility itself. Most facilities do not allow staff members to accept individual tips because they don't want to create a situation where the staff are motivated to care more for certain residents than for others. We believe this is a sound policy. In some states or counties tipping staff members of a nursing home may even be illegal.

Many facilities have a method in place for pooling tips so that all staff members can share in the wealth. This way the people behind the scenes who care for your parent indirectly will get their fair share of the tip, too. If you want to show your appreciation with money, tip your intended amount into the collective pool. Don't try to demonstrate your appreciation to a specific aide by offering money directly to him or her in spite of the institution's no-tipping policy. Being offered a tip "on the sly" can cause conflict for an aide who on the one hand doesn't want to turn down the money, but on the other hand doesn't want to get into trouble for violating policy.

GOOD WAYS TO SHOW YOUR APPRECIATION TO THE STAFF

* Tell them you love the way they care for your parent. (Just don't add the "I couldn't do that" part.)

* Pay attention to their needs and concerns and offer to help when appropriate. If you overhear an aide mentioning that her daughter has asthma and you happen to know a good doctor who specializes in asthma, by all means offer a referral.

* Write a letter or card to the staff as a whole.

* Thank them for their patience.

* If you know your parent has some challenging aspects to his or her personality, reassure the staff that you sympathize with what they are going through—you've been there, too.

* If you are leaving after a visit with a good feeling about the place, say so.

* Find out what they love (chocolate? cookies?) and give it as a gift the whole staff can share.

❋ Give money to the staff tip pool to be split equally among them.

Finally, don't take too much of a staff member's time to show your appreciation. Long conversations about the asthma doctor that you know or about your father's trademark crankiness take your aide away from his or her work with the residents. Give the nursing home staff your honest, positive feedback whenever possible, and it will be much easier to give them negative feedback if it is ever necessary.

Offering Critical Feedback

It is fair to say that even the best nursing homes aren't perfect. At times you may feel that something needs to be changed. You may witness an event that you feel is inappropriate or even dangerous, or you may be concerned about the level of care your parent is receiving. If this is the case, it is vital that you make your feelings known by offering critical feedback to the institution.

Critical feedback can be offered in such a way that it is more likely to be welcomed, heard, received, and acted upon. Feedback can also be offered in such a way that the only thing the recipients can do is to defend themselves against it. In this section we describe the former type. What follows are a few general rules that are worth adhering to if you want your feedback to be as effective as possible. We describe them in the context of a nursing home, but you may find the same principles handy in other situations where you are called upon to provide critical feedback.

1. Give negative feedback as soon as possible. Don't wait until a situation has gone on for so long that you get upset and lose your self-control when you express your concerns.

2. Find out what's really going on before criticizing any situation. Maybe you walked in at 11:00 A.M. and your mom was still in her nightgown. You feel upset and you want to complain. Stay calm and simply ask the staff why your

mother isn't dressed. Maybe she didn't fall asleep until 7:00 A.M. and the staff didn't want to wake her.

3. Never criticize anyone in public.

4. Before you speak with anyone be certain you have made the distinction between the facts of the situation and your feelings about it. When you speak about the matter, if you find yourself using words such as "awful," "terrible," "unacceptable," or any other adjective that conveys judgment, you are talking about your feelings, not about the situation itself. When you have feedback to give to the nursing home staff, stick to the facts and leave the emotional evaluation out of it. "My mother says she was not given any breakfast this morning" will get you much better results than "This is terrible! My mother is being neglected here!"

5. When you speak with the nursing home administrator or any other staff member, take the following steps:

   - Ask to speak privately.

   - Keep your voice respectful and inquiring, not accusatory or attacking.

   - Report exact facts. What did you see? Hear? When? Where?

   - Ask why it happened and who was responsible.

   - Explain why you are concerned.

   - Ask what will be done to correct the problem and to prevent it from happening again.

Can't Get No Satisfaction: What to Do when You Have a Complaint

There are likely to be times when you or your loved one is dissatisfied with a situation in the nursing home. Sometimes this is a problem and sometimes it isn't. Dissatisfaction tends to fall into one of two categories:

1. Habitual dissatisfaction

2. Genuine dissatisfaction

This is true of everyone, including you and your loved one.

HABITUAL DISSATISFACTION

Some people develop a life script in their early years that always includes a certain amount of dissatisfaction. To hear them tell it, they can never lead a wholly satisfied life. Maybe they feel superior or more engaged when they complain. Maybe complaining has become a way of getting attention or manipulating the behavior of others. Or maybe they just stubbornly adhere to a negative way of looking at life (which, humorously enough, such people often describe as being more "realistic" than other points of view).

Whatever a person's reason for embracing such an outlook, it is not dependent on his or her age. Young people can be just as habitually dissatisfied as older people.

Wanda coped very well with all the changes involved in moving to a nursing home. She quickly began taking part in community activities, smiled often, and seemed to enjoy herself. The staff thought she was quite happy overall. Then, after a few weeks, her daughter Penny came back from an extended vacation and visited Wanda for the first time in the nursing home. The administrator was walking through the living room and overheard Wanda complaining bitterly, "Why did you put me in this awful place? They mistreat me terribly. They don't feed me enough. I'm starving here. I don't get enough to eat." Penny became suspicious of the staff, but fortunately she also discovered that her mother's skirt was now too small because her mother had gained several pounds since moving in!

Wanda and Penny were simply playing out a dynamic they had enacted for years. Wanda was no more or less unhappy now than she had ever been; she was simply in the habit of trying to manipulate Penny by complaining. Penny was also a habitually dissatisfied person who usually paid closer attention to her mother's complaints than to any other comments Wanda made. Since her complaints got Penny's attention, Wanda happily supplied them.

Nursing home staff have seen it all. They know that many happy, upbeat, robust residents who stand up straight and walk lively when no one is visiting them will slow their gait, stoop their shoulders, and take on a weak and helpless demeanor when their children arrive. The older people are not necessarily trying to be deceitful; they simply want their children's attention, love, and caring, and they've learned how to get it in some unconscious ways. If you suspect this is the case with your parent, be sure to use your attention and comments to reinforce the behaviors you want to see rather than the ones you don't. If you pay close attention only when your father complains about the staff, don't be surprised if his complaints become more and more frequent and exaggerated.

Studies designed to measure general satisfaction at various stages of life have found that satisfaction in old age relates most closely not to a person's current life but to his or her personality and to the coping techniques he or she learned in the past. If people are satisfied with the life they lived when they were younger, they are much more likely to be content in their old age. If they are unhappy with the way they have lived up until now, their children's jumping through hoops won't improve their satisfaction level today.

GENUINE DISSATISFACTION

But what if your dissatisfaction with the nursing home is based in reality? What if the staff are not responding to your feedback and nothing is changing? The answer to these questions depends on the nature of the complaint and the nature of the facility. Large institutions will probably have a written policy for filing complaints. To get the best results simply read and follow the preferred procedures.

Many smaller institutions rely more on the face-to-face relationship they develop with residents and their families. For your specific issues or complaints to have an impact on the institution as a whole, consider addressing the matter in a meeting of the resident's council or the family member's council (which you will surely want to join). If your loved one's facility doesn't have a family member's council, consider starting one yourself. However, if the problem is more of an isolated situation and doesn't threaten any resident's safety or health, first try the following method.

Find a time when the team leader responsible for your parent's care can pay attention to you. Following the guidelines we provided in the preceding section, let him or her know what the problem is. Submit your complaint in writing whenever possible. Then give the team leader a reasonable amount of time to deal with the situation. If it does not get resolved in what you consider a fair amount of time, ask the team leader why the situation hasn't changed. If you don't get satisfaction from the team leader, and depending on what the issue is, next you can address your complaint to the head nurse or to the nursing home director or administrator.

For example, if the bulb in your father's bedside reading lamp is burned out, let the team leader know about it. If it's still burned out a week later, you may need to talk to the director. If a month goes by and the bulb still has not been changed, you will want to talk to the director again. This time, your conversation may be about more than just the bulb. You may also want to indicate that you are losing confidence in the nursing home because of their lack of responsiveness. What would happen, you may wonder aloud, if the complaint was of a more serious nature?

Of course, if the complaint is a safety issue, see that it is taken care of immediately. Suppose, for example, that you are visiting your mother and you notice some fresh scratches on her roommate's arm. When you ask the aide what happened, she shrugs and says, "Nothing." The next day you notice more scratches on the woman's other arm. This time you ask the team leader about it. Since you are not the woman's relative you may not be entitled to know what is happening, but a good team leader can and will reassure you that the staff is aware of the problem and that, although they can't discuss the details with you, they are taking measures to prevent it from happening again. A not-so-good team leader will dismiss your complaint and leave you feeling unheard. In that case, it's a good idea to go immediately to the director or, depending on the severity of the situation, to an outside agency. Most states have a government agency that is responsible for dealing with nursing home complaints. California, for example, has a state ombudsman devoted to long-term-care issues. Check out longtermcarelink.net, a website that contains links to the sites of many state agencies providing senior services and nursing home oversight. In addition, many support groups and organizations, such as WISE Senior Services, in Los Angeles, can advise you about how best to proceed from a legal standpoint. See the Resources for contact information for both of these organizations.

Now that you know how to work with the staff, you are prepared to get the most from the nursing home environment. There are only a few more things you need to know. We tell you all about them in the next chapter.

Chapter 12

Other Important Things to Know

This chapter is a compilation of topics we think you'll want and need to be informed about. The subjects addressed are those most frequently asked about by family members or most often featured in the media. In this chapter we cover the following:

* Dehydration

* Addictions

* Dementia (read this even if your loved one is not suffering from dementia)

* Sexuality

* Laundry complaints

* Money (under the resident's control)

* Housekeeping

* The use of restraints

* Changing institutions

* Leaving the nursing home

Dehydration

If your parent seems confused, unfocused, or inattentive when you visit, it may be because of the medication he or she is taking, it may be due a neurological condition, or it may be the result of dehydration. Dehydration, or not drinking enough fluids, is a common problem for nursing home residents and a common point of focus for the staff. In past generations no one paid much attention to how much water older (or younger) people drank, but in recent years we have learned much more about the importance of drinking enough fluids. We now know how much water people need to consume to stay healthy, and nursing home staff members are aware of the importance of encouraging residents to drink as much as possible.

Unfortunately, elderly people sometimes lose (or have never fully developed) their natural sense of thirst. In addition, most of today's nursing home residents were not raised with the notion that it was important to drink much water. To them, staying well hydrated is simply unimportant. Sometimes they refuse to drink as much as the health professionals think is necessary, or sometimes they are simply too weak to raise a glass to their lips. Imagine being a nursing home aide. You hand Mrs. Miller a cup of water and encourage her to drink. Verrrry slooooowly, Mrs. Miller takes the cup. She gradually lifts it to her lips. She takes a tiny sip, and she thanks you for the drink. Mrs. Miller feels she has had quite enough to drink. You know she ideally needs to drink ten full cups each day—but that is simply not going to happen.

Although nursing home staff members are very aware of the dangers of dehydration, they also know how inhumane it would be to force residents to drink far more than the residents want to drink. To compensate, nursing homes serve a lot of fluid-based foods, such as soups, creamy yogurts, and juices—but rarely do today's nursing home residents consume what doctors would consider "enough" fluids. Sometimes nursing homes are forced to bolster a resident's hydration levels with an intravenous drip, just to restore the resident's strength for the time being.

As a special note, if your parent is taking a diuretic drug to remove fluids from his or her lungs or joints or heart, it may seem as though your parent should drink less water, not more, but exactly the opposite is true. If your mother's or father's medication removes fluids from the body, your parent will need to consume even more than the recommended eight to ten glasses of water per day to stay healthy and alert.

Addictions

If your parent suffers from an addiction, find out what the facility's policy is toward his or her particular case. Most nursing homes embrace a tolerant attitude toward addictions that are the result of decades-old habits. They don't want the resident to feel deprived, so they do their best to provide what is necessary for his or her comfort. The most common addictions that nursing home residents arrive with are addictions to

* alcohol
* tobacco
* food
* prescription drugs

ALCOHOL

Your parent may not be an alcoholic, but some people are. There are likely to be several residents in your loved one's nursing home who are there due to alcoholism-related diseases. In some cases, as the resident reaches old age and his or her condition progresses, tolerance may decrease and the desire for a drink may decrease along with it. Others are still addicted and may lose self-control and get aggressive unless they have enough to drink each day. These residents may be allowed to receive a certain quantity of alcohol each day to maintain a basic level of self-control, for example, three or four beers.

What is more dangerous and is somewhat common is the kind of hidden alcoholism that some residents have developed in old age. Many residents arrive at a nursing home after having lived alone for some time. They may have gradually, and quietly, increased their alcohol consumption over the years as a form of self-medication to ward off depression and feelings of isolation. They usually deny the addiction. Once in the nursing home they may switch from alcohol to a sedating medication such as sleeping pills, and they may be very aggressive or depressed without knowing exactly why. If the nursing home staff suspects an addiction of this type, they may work with you to help your loved one gradually reduce his or her alcohol consumption. Eventually the love, attention, and activity in the nursing home may come to replace your parent's loneliness-related drinking.

FOOD

Food addictions are common among members of today's older generation. Many people who are now over seventy went through hard times when they were younger. Whether their deprivation resulted from Depression-era economics, living in a war-torn region, or being born into a poverty-stricken immigrant family, many current nursing home residents knew hunger at some time during their formative years. People who have been traumatized by hunger may develop a hoarding mentality toward food. They may never feel as though they have enough. Even when they can see that food is now plentiful, some people still fear that it will all be gone tomorrow.

Nursing homes are generally tolerant of food addictions, and as long as residents' food choices are medically safe, residents are allowed to eat as much as they like of whatever they want. For the most part, residents who are psychologically addicted to food may find themselves restricted more by diabetes or the simple loss of appetite that often occurs in old age than by nursing home policy.

MEDICATION

When residents arrive at a nursing home, they may be on their way to an addiction to sleeping pills, sedating medications such as Valium, or pain medication. They may have been self-medicating with over-the-counter drugs, or they may have received prescription therapies that have continued longer than necessary. Nursing home staff will do their best to determine whether an addiction is physical or psychological and will also try to determine whether the addiction itself is problematic enough to warrant the discomfort a patient will go through if eased off the drug in question. Sometimes the addiction will be allowed to continue if the drug is not otherwise harming the patient. It can be especially difficult to say no to someone who is addicted to a pain medication because the perception of pain is very personal and the resident may actually be suffering.

Nursing home staff will work to reduce an addiction problem while still maintaining the resident's comfort as best they can. Sometimes a resident's frequent requests for medication are a way of seeking attention. In such cases a simple placebo, such as an M&M candy, dispensed by the nurse, often has the same effect as the medication.

TOBACCO

Tobacco can be the strongest addiction of all. Even people who are sentenced to death often request one last cigarette. Nursing home residents who smoke are often heard to say, "I have nothing else to live for but my cigarettes," or, "I have no joy in life but my cigarettes." Nursing homes can't really forbid an addicted smoker from smoking. The resident may agree not to, but he or she will usually still try to sneak cigarettes, which makes for a dangerous situation. If a resident is weak or unsteady or drowsy, he or she needs close supervision while smoking to avoid a serious fire hazard. Most nursing homes offer supervised smoking areas for residents.

Whether or not your parent is a smoker, be sure to find out how your nursing home deals with residents who do smoke. Simply having a blanket no-smoking policy is insufficient, as it will drive the smokers underground, and that's dangerous.

Dementia

Many nursing homes have some residents who are suffering from dementia of one type or another. Your parent may not be one of them, but chances are both you and your parent will have contact with them. Residents with dementia may repeatedly ask you (or your parent) what time it is or what day it is, or they may take your parent's coffee because they don't know that it isn't theirs. You may have a hard time understanding their speech, or they may approach you thinking that you are their spouse or child. Be friendly, and don't be aggressive. If you feel embarrassed or intruded upon by the presence of residents with dementia, you may want to arrange to meet your parent elsewhere.

Dementia patients are not like children. They may have a childlike way of relating to the world, but there is one very important difference to keep in mind. Most dementia patients still retain their emotional sense of memory. When they soil their diapers, they may not understand why, but they may feel shame. When they encounter someone who is frowning or speaking harshly to them, they may not understand what is happening, but they will know enough to feel hurt or frightened. Be kind and patient and respectful, and remember that even though it may not be your parent who is asking you what time it is every five minutes, it is probably somebody's mother or father.

Sexuality

There were times when nursing home floors were segregated by sex. Even married couples could not stay in the same room. At least nursing homes were acknowledging older people as sexual beings. Later, coed floors were introduced, an indication of the belief that older people were "harmless" and basically not sexual at all. Nowadays, whether or not active sexuality between residents is accepted depends on the philosophy of the institution.

Ask about your nursing home's policy. Each home bases its rules on its own orientation and cultural background. Some frown upon any sexual contact between residents, while others take a more tolerant approach. Special-interest homes are beginning to be available for gay, lesbian, and transgender seniors. It is never appropriate for an institution to tolerate sexual contact between staff members and residents.

Regardless of how tolerant a nursing home may be of sexual expression, many diseases and medications of old age reduce the libido to the point where sexuality is no longer an issue. Still, plenty of love affairs spring up between affectionate, hand-holding residents, and requests for privacy between residents are quite normal. When Grandma suddenly starts rediscovering her body, it is usually far more astonishing to the family members than it is to the staff or other residents.

Laundry Complaints (or, Nobody Is Stealing Your Mother's Underwear)

Missing laundry is a common source of conflict in nursing homes. For some practical tips to help prevent lost clothing, review the section in Chapter 7 about preparing clothing for the nursing home. In addition, be aware that even the most refined system of labeling and identifying laundry cannot guarantee that items will never go astray. Avoid buying expensive clothing for your mother or father. And before you respond by getting upset and making a scene, think about whether it's really a worthwhile expenditure of your life energy to yell at an aide about a missing sweater.

If your parent seems low on clean clothes, ask whether you have brought enough. Maybe your parent has had diarrhea and his or her clothes needed to be changed more often than usual. Or maybe some clothes have worn out and need to be replaced. If more than one or two pieces of laundry per month actually do go missing, they should be replaced by the laundry company. Talk to the team leader responsible for your loved one's care. The best strategy is to write down your complaint and include a list of missing items and the approximate dates they disappeared.

Sometimes items will go missing because of a problem with the nursing home's distribution system. Maybe the aide assigned to return laundry couldn't read well or made a simple mistake. Perhaps the aide fails to realize that he or she needs to wear his or her glasses when sorting the laundry. A good nursing home will appreciate knowing when internal mistakes occur. Be sure to use diplomacy and respect when reporting such errors. Regardless of how you handle the situation, there is one thing you can be sure of: Nobody is stealing your mother's underwear.

Money

When a nursing home resident has money in his pocket it gives him a feeling of security and importance, even if he is suffering from dementia. Normally each resident's room contains a special locker in which to store things of value. But what if your mother forgets to lock it, or she loses her key, or she simply doesn't want to bother using it? When money goes missing, the staff hears the question frequently asked by nursing home residents everywhere: "Who has stolen my money?"

Before we cover how to handle valuables, let's address the following question:

HOW MUCH MONEY SHOULD BE AT THE RESIDENT'S DISPOSAL?

Whenever possible, the resident should have control over his or her own money. But even most residents who don't pay their own bills want to have a certain amount of pocket money available, which they will probably keep in their room. How much money your parent has at his or her disposal depends on the situation. It should only be as much as your parent can afford to lose without catastrophe. For one person that's a thousand dollars, and for another it's ten dollars.

Your loved one may have opportunities to purchase items at the nursing home. Perhaps there is a cafeteria or food mart on the premises. Or your parent may want to pay for a taxi, go shopping, attend outings and excursions, or purchase special services, such as hair styling or a massage. Some residents may feel anxious if they don't think they can pay for things.

Residents with dementia sometimes grow agitated at mealtime if they don't believe they can pay for their dinner, no matter how much the aides reassure them that they will not be charged. Having even a few coins in their purse or pocket can help them feel much better. Somehow it makes everything okay. The aides will usually tell them that they can pay for their food later.

Of course, sometimes the other extreme can occur.

Eric, age ninety-eight, was a little senile, but he didn't suffer from dementia. He simply preferred to live in the past. One day, a volunteer, a rather attractive young woman, leaned over Eric to fill his coffee, and he slipped a hundred-dollar bill into her bra! It was his way of showing appreciation, and it allowed him to feel important and respected.

HOW TO HANDLE VALUABLES

If you can't be sure that valuable or sentimental possessions are secure in your parent's room, or that your parent can handle a locker and key, be sure to store them somewhere else. Some facilities have central lockers where small precious items such as jewelry and money can be kept. If the item is really special, take it home with you. You can't prevent your mother from inviting someone into her room who may suffer from dementia. Residents who don't know what belongs to them will often take interesting little things without really intending to steal them.

Housekeeping

When you visit your parent's nursing home, you may expect it to look like a brochure, with smiling, clean residents engaged in fulfilling activities and wearing appreciative expressions on their faces. We are quite sure there are institutions out there that look just like the architectural drawings—spotless and perfect—but we haven't found them yet.

Perhaps you have lived with small children. If so, you may remember the rather large messes that attended their most joyful and creative moments. At times maybe you felt wistfully envious of the neighbor down the block who always had floors so clean you could eat off of them, but somehow you knew that life was an exciting, chaotic force that was often downright messy. In or out of a nursing home, there is a parallel between living in a relaxed way and living comfortably. You may walk into your mother's facility and see a newspaper on the living room floor. The chairs may be askew and the sofa cushions piled awkwardly. These are signs of life in a nursing home.

Of course, we're not talking about accepting unsanitary conditions. There is no good excuse for old dirt caked in the corners, or dust-covered windowsills, but the nursing home that shows some untidiness will undoubtedly be a happier and more comfortable place to live than a sterile, orderly, magazine-perfect environment. We would even go so far as to value a warm, relaxed, and loving atmosphere above perfectly clean conditions. If you feel comfortable in your parent's nursing home but you happen to notice some dirt caked in the corner, perhaps this is an opportunity for you to help the facility find a good housekeeper. Nursing home administrators are not perfect. They are called upon to be experts in many different areas. They need to possess medical knowledge, people skills, and management expertise. Housekeeping skills are important, but all of these qualities may not coexist in equal measures in the same person.

You may remember Athena, the businesswoman from Chapters 4 and 5. When her mother, Anna, fell and needed care, Athena automatically assumed that Anna would come home to live with her and her husband, Joe. Instead, Anna shocked Athena by insisting on moving into a facility near her own home.

Athena was livid the first time she visited Anna in her new home. Anna seemed happy enough, but in Athena's opinion the place was filthy—and she loudly made her feelings known to the staff. Athena was looking for things to complain about. She was still hoping to convince her mother to live with her and Joe. She believed that if she pointed out the facility's flaws, Anna would agree that things were horrible and would change her mind about living there.

But Anna remained firm and refused to leave. Athena went home feeling miserable. The next day, in her weekly therapy session, Athena mentioned her feelings to Mark, her therapist. Mark asked Athena what was most troubling to her about Anna's living in a nursing home. Athena responded, "The place is filthy! You can barely see out the windows because they are so dirty!"

Mark suggested that Athena consider cleaning the windows at the facility if that was all that was bothering her. Athena was stunned. She didn't know what to say. But after thinking about Mark's advice for several weeks, she decided to give it a try. On her next visit to Anna's nursing home, Athena arrived with bucket, sponge, and squeegee in hand.

At first her attitude was hostile. "I'll show them how this is supposed to be done," she thought. But as she rolled up her sleeves and got busy, something happened. Several residents came over and watched. Some asked her questions. Others offered window-cleaning advice. Even the home's director came by and introduced himself. Everyone seemed happy to see her there. Anna, looking happiest of all, watched her daughter from the sofa. Athena's attitude about the place started to change.

That incident took place several years ago. Anna still lives there, and now Athena is a member of the institution's board of directors. She regularly puts her management and business skills to work for a good cause, as she makes sure her mother and the other residents are well looked after.

If your nursing home director is gifted at providing a loving, safe, and warm environment, but is a bit weak in the area of housekeeping, perhaps you could see it as an opportunity to be of service. Consider gently (and respectfully) offering your help. Offering to help is usually a better choice than choosing to get frustrated and causing a stir, or moving to the cleaner but colder place down the block.

DIRTY CLOTHING

If you are a frequent visitor to your parent's nursing home, you'll soon have a sense of the facility's laundry schedule. You'll notice whether stains from food or other causes appear frequently or occasionally on your parent's clothing. But if you visit once a month or less often, you may be dismayed to see your parent wearing an item of clothing that looks unclean. There are several possible reasons why this can happen:

* Neglect

* Economics

* Love

Neglect: If you suspect that your mother's stained cardigan is a sign of neglect, look around. Some institutions really do neglect their residents. If this is the case, your mother's sweater won't be the only sign of a pattern of neglect. Reread Chapter 6 to learn the other signs of neglect, and keep an eye out for them. If neglect seems a likely culprit, you can complain to the team leader or the director, using the suggestions in Chapter 11. If the signs are severe, you may decide to move your parent to another facility.

Economics: Many nursing homes work hard to keep costs down. If they didn't, most facilities would be far too expensive for the average person to afford. One way to cut costs is to do laundry every other day rather than daily. That means sometimes a garment will be worn twice before it gets washed. If cost-cutting measures are behind the stains on your father's vest, consider the severity of the situation. A little ketchup on his lapel may not be all that serious. Yet incontinence residue on his pants should never be tolerated, and a sweater that had water spilled on it should be changed quickly so he doesn't get chilled.

Love: In a close relationship, feeding another person can be an act of intimacy, love, and caring. But being fed by a stranger as a matter of functionality can be very uncomfortable. It does not allow the person who is eating to chew and swallow comfortably at his or her own pace, and it can feel very demeaning. In the best nursing homes, residents are allowed and expected to do as much for themselves as they possibly can, not because of a lack of caring, but as a sign of respect for each resident's abilities. If your mother can still feed herself, even if she's rather messy about it, she will probably be encouraged to do so. And if she spills a few drops of food on her dress while she eats, it is often more humane for the staff to look the other way than it would be for them to humiliate her by insisting that she wear a bib, or that she change her dress immediately because she has soiled it.

There are other reasons why your loved one's clothing may be soiled.

Will was eighty-two when he moved into a nursing home after living on his own for several years. He suffered from extreme vertigo and could no longer drive, shop, cook, or care for himself. Will had a fine wardrobe of trousers, but he refused to let the laundry service have his favorite "lucky" pants. Day after day, Will wore those pants in spite of the staff's pleading and urging. Will often spilled food on himself, so the pants showed a full menu of what he had eaten over the last several weeks. He was also a little incontinent, so the pants were more than a bit aromatic, too. The smell didn't bother Will, just everyone around him. But no matter how bad they got, Will would not allow his lucky pants to be cleaned.

The staff discussed the matter of Will's lucky pants in a meeting and came up with a creative solution. Twice a week, the night nurse quietly removed Will's pants from his room, laundered them herself, and returned them to him before he woke up in the morning. Will never noticed that his pants had been cleaned. As long as they were there in the morning, he was happy.

Before you complain to the staff about your mother's spotted blouse or your father's nasty trousers, be sure to get a full understanding of what is really behind the mess.

The Use of Restraints

Restraints are an emotional topic, and as a result there is a great deal of misinformation about their use. The media often report that a nursing home has used restraints to tie older people into their beds or wheelchairs in inhumane ways. Whenever we hear about such a case, it is easy to identify with the resident, which can cause us to feel terrible. In fact, it is illegal to restrain a resident simply for the convenience of the nursing home staff. Use of restraints for this reason is a crime and should be immediately prosecuted.

However, some types of restraints are both humane and necessary for the protection and safety of nursing home residents. Restraints fall into two categories: chemical restraints (consisting of sedating drugs), and physical restraints, such as bedrails, wheelchair tables that cannot be opened by the resident, incontinence suits that the resident cannot take off (to keep residents with dementia from relieving themselves in various inappropriate locations around the facility), and belts used to keep a resident from falling out of a bed or wheelchair.

Restraints are only for the protection of the resident. Some residents are very weak or cannot control their muscular movements. They need to be restrained in their wheelchair or bed so they do not fall out. Others may simply forget that they cannot walk or that they have severe vertigo. They may try to get up and walk if not properly restrained.

There is no excuse for the improper use of restraints, but there are several proper uses for them. Be sure you are involved in the discussion and permission process if the use of restraints is advised in the care of your parent. Develop a good understanding of the reasons behind any need for restraints, and if you are still suspicious about their necessity, call your state's long-term-care ombudsman (see Resources).

Changing Institutions

Once your parent is living in a nursing home, there may come a time when you decide it would be best to leave the facility for another living arrangement. This can happen for several reasons:

Your parent is dissatisfied. If your mother or father seems unhappy with the current nursing home, do your best to determine if the dissatisfaction is based in reality or if it is part of a pattern of habitual dissatisfaction. If the dissatisfaction is genuine and cannot be rectified in the current facility, perhaps a change is in order. On the other hand, if the dissatisfaction is the result of habitual crankiness, moving to another facility is unlikely to make much of a difference.

The grass is greener. Perhaps a room in the beautiful new nursing home across town has just opened up. You've been on the waiting list since the place was under construction. It has lovely gardens and wonderful views. You're considering jumping at the chance to move your parent there. Or maybe you've been promoted at work and transferred to a different city. You're thinking of taking your parent with you and moving him or her into a nursing home in the new town.

Before you make the change, it is important to stop and ask yourself a few questions:

* Has your parent made friends where he or she is now?

* Has your parent gotten acquainted with the staff members in the current home?

* Even if your parent complains about some aspects of the place, is he or she generally integrated and involved in community life there?

✴ Did it take your parent a while to adjust to the current environment?

If you answered yes to any of these questions, you may want to seriously consider leaving your parent where he or she is. Moving is stressful under any circumstances, but it is more stressful for older people. Their bodies are weaker. They have to spend their limited energy learning the layout of a new building, getting to know their fellow residents, and developing trust with the people who will help them perform their most intimate physical tasks. Just as transplanting a young oak tree is a rather simple task, while moving an old oak tree will likely kill it, moving your parent unnecessarily can cause him or her extreme stress and trauma.

If your parent is unaware of his or her surroundings or has not integrated into the community, you'll have to use your best judgment about whether he or she can physically handle a move. Seek the advice of your parent's doctor if you are unsure.

You or your spouse has retired, and you feel you can now take care of your parent at home. It is becoming increasingly common for the adult children of nursing home residents to reach retirement age themselves. If this is your situation, you may believe that retirement will afford you the necessary time and energy to care for your parent at home. Before you decide, please review Chapter 4, "The Home-Care Instinct," to get a good sense of what home care is like. After giving the matter careful thought, if you sincerely believe you can handle it, if your parent agrees to the move, if your reasons for wanting to do it are clear and honest, and if your relationship with your parent has been a good one for a long time—by all means, take your parent home. But please be very sure you've thought through all the above issues before making the move. It will be stressful on your parent to move in with you and adjust to a new life, probably one offering less stimulation, but it will be even more stressful if things don't work out and you have to return your parent to the nursing home a few months later.

If you and your parent decide to leave a facility, for whatever reason, be sure to familiarize yourself with the relevant aspects of the agreement you signed when moving your parent in. Every facility has its own departure policies, but most require cancellation in writing and with a certain amount of notice. You'll probably be required to pay the fees through the end of the month regardless of when your parent actually leaves, but some facilities may offer a discount for days when the resident doesn't eat meals or have laundry done.

One last point bears mentioning. Perhaps your father entered the nursing home with the ability to negotiate and sign his own admissions contract. Maybe in the intervening months his mental abilities have deteriorated to where he no longer can take care of such business. If this is the case, be certain that you are legally entitled to renegotiate the agreement he entered into when he was of sound mind. The laws vary from state to state, so be sure to seek professional guidance in this matter.

If your parent is still of sound mind, you may want to discuss with him or her the possibility of drafting a durable power of attorney. A durable power of attorney is a legal document specifying who is responsible for handling a person's financial and legal affairs if that person becomes incapacitated. We strongly advise you to have these sorts of discussions with your parents while they are still able to participate willingly. Doing so makes things much easier later on.

Saying Goodbye: Leaving the Nursing Home

Sooner or later, your mother or father will leave the nursing home. Occasionally a resident's health or abilities may improve as the result of therapy, and the resident is able to return to his or her own home or to move into an assisted-living facility. Sometimes a resident has a health crisis that requires a trip to the hospital. And sometimes residents naturally come to the end of their lives in the nursing home. Regardless of how your parent leaves the nursing home, there will come a time to say goodbye to his or her friends and "adopted" family there.

LEAVING THE NURSING HOME TO GO HOME

Sometimes people feel so good after a period of time in a nursing home that they want to go home. They think they are well and can return to normal life. They may fail to take into account how much is being done for them in the nursing home. As was the case with Xenia's mother, after a few days or weeks at home they often realize how much energy it takes to do their own laundry or cook their own meals, and they decide to return to the nursing home for good.

In other cases, a son or daughter decides to take the resident home to live with him or her.

> Sumi was in her early nineties and had to be looked after twenty-four hours a day. When her daughter Aki retired from her job as a schoolteacher, she decided to bring her mother into her home. It was a pleasure for Aki to spend time with Sumi. The two had always enjoyed a close relationship, and now they could spend their days together. Aki hired a housekeeper and spent her time taking her mother on walks and excursions around town.

LEAVING THE NURSING HOME TO GO TO ASSISTED LIVING

Sometimes residents' health improves during their stay in a nursing home. They may choose to move into an assisted-living facility.

> Gladys was sent to a nursing home after a hospital stay. She arrived with a severe case of pneumonia, and she also suffered from disorientation. After three months in the nursing home Gladys was back to her old self, feeling strong and mentally sound. She no longer needed nursing care, but she decided she did not want to go back to living by herself because she was tired of doing her own shopping and housework, and she didn't want to risk wearing herself out and getting sick again.

Gladys moved into an assisted-living facility located across the street from the nursing home. She still drives, and is currently traveling abroad, but her plants are being watered and she needn't worry about who is shoveling the snow in the driveway. She says, "I like knowing that I am part of a community of people who care for me. Why would I ever want to live all alone again?"

LEAVING THE NURSING HOME TO GO TO THE HOSPITAL

When a resident leaves the nursing home to go to the hospital, the journey may be one way or round trip, and it may be for a long time or just a short while. Regardless of how long your loved one stays in the hospital, it is their right to keep their room at the nursing home, and it is also their duty to continue paying for it. If you would like to cancel your mother's or father's room at the home, be sure to follow the institution's policies.

PASSING AWAY IN A NURSING HOME

Most people in nursing homes are either old or very old. Since everyone dies, to some extent the death of a nursing home resident is often expected. That's not to say that the death of a parent is ever an easy or pleasant time, just that there are certain situations in which it is to be expected. We wish to make a few points about nursing homes and death.

Not a place to die, a place to live. There are a lot of people, books, and techniques that can tell you how someone should die. We don't favor any one of these theories over another. We believe that people are simply living their lives right up until their last moments, and that death is just a natural part of life. Even if your parent or other loved one is in a nursing home to spend the last remaining portion of his or her life, we suggest doing your best to think of those final days as a part of your loved one's life, as much as any other. As long as people are alive, they are alive, no matter what that looks like.

Family members will encounter death in a nursing home. Everyone who enters a nursing home is confronted with death in one way or another. You may see people who already look as though they are dead because they are lying in bed unconscious and barely breathing. You may visit one day and notice that someone is "missing." Where is the little old lady who used to sit in the corner and knit? One day she just isn't there anymore. "In memoriam" notices about residents who have died may be posted on the community bulletin boards. The point we're making is that nobody can predict when a nursing home resident (or anyone else) will die.

Practices and philosophies about death. Be sure you know the answers to the following questions about your nursing home's policies:

* Are you allowed to stay overnight in the nursing home with your dying family member?

* What happens if your loved one is dying in a shared room?

* Does your nursing home offer hospice-style care (see below)?

* What happens after death has occurred?

Some facilities move a dying person to the hospital to die there, and others allow them to pass more naturally in their own nursing "home," if that is what the resident desires. Many facilities can do either, depending upon the wishes of the resident and his or her family members.

Nursing homes and hospice care. Hospice care is a philosophical alternative to regular hospital care. It originated as an option for people who are terminally ill and fairly close to death. The word "hospice" is often used to mean a particular type of facility, but the hospice philosophy toward the end of life can be practiced anywhere and by anyone. Hospice care can be provided within a hospital setting, in a special hospice unit, at the patient's home, or in a nursing home, depending upon the availability of care, the philosophy of the institution, and the special needs of the patient. Hospice care is designed to make the last period of a person's life as worthwhile as possible. It provides a completely different atmosphere from a traditional hospital stay. Some hospice workers are skilled health-care professionals and others are caring volunteers. Depending on the setting, a patient in hospice care can enjoy his or her favorite meals as well as other things he or she likes, can visit with his or her pets, and can receive as much pain relief as he or she requests.

Your parent's nursing home may practice a hospice-style approach to dying by trying to make the dying resident as comfortable as possible. This may mean giving a diabetic resident a piece of candy if he or she asks for it, or honoring an alcoholic's request for a drink. Or the facility may take the opposite approach and move dying residents to a traditional hospital setting to try to prolong their lives. Some facilities will do either, depending upon the resident's and the family's preferences, so be sure to let the administrators know what your personal choices are and ask if the staff can honor them.

Make your wishes known in advance. In some cases, there are indications that death is approaching. You can discuss in advance with the team leader whether you want to be called if your parent exhibits any such signs. Be sure to make your wishes known. Nursing home administrators cannot guess what your preferences might be in such a situation.

What happens after death has occurred? Ask how death is handled in your particular institution. Sometimes death simply doesn't fit into the image the nursing home wants to project, and the body and all personal effects must be removed from the facility as quickly as possible. In other places, you may sit with your deceased loved one and hold a vigil that corresponds with your spiritual, religious, or cultural beliefs.

Special Goodbyes

THE SUITCASE

Maggie was a ninety-three-year-old former schoolteacher who had lived in her nursing home for more than two years. The staff remembers her as being like a beautiful, old-fashioned doll. She had never been married and was a devoted Catholic. She had a huge old suitcase in her room. No one knew what was in that suitcase. Maggie told everyone they could not open it until the day she died. The staff often tried to guess what was in it, but Maggie would never tell.

One night Maggie died peacefully in her sleep. The nursing home staff went into mourning, because everybody loved Maggie, but their grief was mixed with curiosity about what was in the mysterious suitcase. The morning after her death, the staff gathered in her room and the nursing home director opened the suitcase. Everyone leaned forward to see what was inside. There, carefully folded and wrapped in tissue paper, was a beautiful, old-fashioned wedding dress. It had clearly never been worn. An envelope contained written instructions in Maggie's handwriting. She wanted to be buried in the wedding dress. She had saved herself all her life for this moment, when she believed she would become a bride of Christ. She wanted to appear in heaven dressed in all her wedding splendor.

GRATITUDE AND FORGIVENESS

Greta was ninety-eight years old and dying, but she wasn't doing it peacefully. She was struggling and straining and screaming against the inevitable. She had kept herself alive for weeks beyond what the doctors had anticipated. After sitting at her mother's bedside watching Greta resist for days, her daughter Laura, age sixty, was exhausted. It seemed as though Greta simply would not let go.

That night at home, Laura prayed for her mother's peaceful release from suffering. She was saying the Lord's Prayer when suddenly she was struck with a realization of what the prayer was about. It was about expressing gratitude, asking for forgiveness, and offering forgiveness to others. As soon as Laura had that awareness, she expressed her gratitude for her mother, asked for her forgiveness, and offered her own forgiveness for Greta's mistakes. Just then, the telephone rang. It was the nursing home calling. Greta had finally relaxed and died peacefully, just as Laura was hoping she would.

GOING "HOME" TO DIE

Bonnie was a sixty-seven-year-old resident of Mountain View Nursing Home. She had been sober for more than eight years, but her physical health had been destroyed by her earlier alcohol abuse. One day Bonnie grew quite ill and had to be moved to the hospital. When it became clear that she was dying, she asked to leave the hospital. She told the doctor she wanted to go home to die.

Since Bonnie had two grown daughters, the doctor naturally assumed that Bonnie meant she wanted to spend her last days in one of their homes. But Bonnie set her straight. "I want to go back to Mountain View," she insisted. "That is my home. Here in the hospital I'm only a case. At Mountain View, I'm a human being."

Bonnie was transferred back to her nursing home, where she died peacefully two days later.

THE BICYCLE AND THE LLAMA'S WOOL COAT

The relationships forged between nursing home staff members and residents can become very close. Sometimes they continue even beyond the death of the resident.

Hanna was eighty-seven when she went to live in the nursing home in her small rural town. For nearly forty years Hanna had worked as the housekeeper for Dr. Belkin, the only doctor in the area. Dr. Belkin was a kind woman who treated the townspeople at her house, so everyone in the area came to know Hanna as the woman who greeted them at the doctor's door and showed them into the study to wait.

Hanna was very proud of her position as Dr. Belkin's housekeeper, and the doctor took good care of Hanna. One year the doctor gave Hanna a beautiful new bicycle to ride to work. Hanna loved that bicycle and rode it everywhere. On another occasion Dr. Belkin gave Hanna an exquisite coat made from llama's wool. Hanna could frequently be seen riding her bicycle through the town while wearing the coat.

In the nursing home, Hanna reminisced often about the good doctor, her wonderful bicycle, and her precious coat. "Have you seen my bicycle?" she would ask. "It's one of the best bicycles ever made. Dr. Belkin gave it to me, you know. And have you seen my coat? It's llama's wool. Very rare. Dr. Belkin gave it to me. I'm sure you have never seen one quite like it."

Hanna had never married or had children. When she died, her body was cremated and her ashes placed in an unmarked county grave. But the nursing home staff wanted to do something more. They loved Hanna and they knew that the townspeople loved her too. So the nursing home paid for an announcement in the newspaper and hosted a memorial service at a local church. More than two hundred people showed up to pay their last respects to Hanna. On display were her famous bicycle and the wonderful llama's wool coat.

In Conclusion

❧ ❧ ❧

Reading this book has provided you with an opportunity to see nursing homes through new lenses. We hope that we have helped to dispel any fears and misconceptions you may have held about long-term care. We hope that you can now envision nursing homes as the caring places they are, where people are accepted regardless of their condition and are provided with enough assistance and compassion to allow them to live with dignity.

We trust that what you've read here has equipped you to take responsibility for making your own or your loved one's long-term-care experience as positive as possible, and that you feel empowered to do so. If living in a nursing home ever becomes a necessity for you or a loved one, we hope that the information provided here can help you feel better—or even good—about the situation.

We'd love to hear from you. Please feel free to write to us about your long-term-care experiences, and to let us know what you think of the book. We can be reached through our publisher:

Lynn Dickinson or Xenia Vosen
c/o Hunter House Publishers
PO Box 2914
Alameda CA 94501

Recommended Reading

❧ ❧ ❧

Alson, Sheila, and Burnett, Gayle. *Peace in Everyday Relationships.* Alameda, CA: Hunter House Publishers, 2003.

Bourne, E.; Garano, L.; and Bourne, E. *Coping with Anxiety: 10 Simple Ways to Relieve Anxiety, Fear, and Worry.* Oakland, CA: New Harbinger Publications, 2003.

Davis, Ruth. *The Nursing Home Handbook.* Holbrook, MA: Adams Media, 1999.

Goleman, Daniel. *Emotional Intelligence: Why It Can Matter More than IQ.* New York: Bantam, 1997.

Johnson, S., and Blanchard, K. *Who Moved My Cheese? An Amazing Way to Deal with Change in Your Work and in Your Life.* New York: Penguin Putnam, 1998.

Morris, Virginia. *How to Care for Aging Parents.* New York: Workman Publishing, 1996.

Pipher, Mary. *Another Country: Navigating the Emotional Terrain of our Elders.* New York: Riverhead Books, 1999.

Ruiz, Don Miguel. *The Four Agreements.* San Rafael, CA: Amber-Allen Publishing, 1997.

Williams, Mark E., M.D. *The American Geriatric Society's Complete Guide to Aging and Health.* New York: Harmony, 1995.

Bibliography

❧ ❧ ❧

American Lung Association, Research and Scientific Affairs Epidemiology and Statistics Unit. *Trends in Pneumonia and Influenza Morbidity and Mortality*. August 2004.

Applebaum, Robert A.; Mehdizadeh, Shahla A.; and Stroker, Jane K. "The Changing World of Long-Term Care: A State Perspective." *Journal of Aging and Social Policy* 16(1): 1–19, 2004.

Billig, N. *Growing Older and Wiser: Coping with Expectations, Challenges, and Change in the Later Years*. New Britain, CT: Lexington Books, 1993.

Binstock, R.H., and George, L.K., eds. *Handbook of Aging and the Social Sciences*, 3rd ed. New York: Academic Press, 1990.

Brock, D.B.; Guralnik, J.M.; and Brody, J.A. "Demography and Epidemiology of Aging in the United States." From *Handbook of the Biology of Aging*, 3rd ed., Schneider, E.L., and Rowe, J.W., eds. New York: Academic Press, 1990, 3–23.

Bury, Michael, and Holme, Andrea. *Life after Ninety*. London and New York: Routledge, 1991.

Capsi, A., and Elder, G.H., Jr. "Life Satisfaction in Old Age: Linking Social Psychology and History." *Psychology and Aging* (1): 18–26, Mar. 1986.

Eckert, Kevin; Morgan, Leslie A.; and Suramy, Namratha. "Preferences for Receipt of Care among Community-Dwelling Adults." *Journal of Aging and Social Policy* 16(2): 49–65, 2004.

"Geographic Profile of the Aged." *Statistical Bulletin* 74(1): 2–9, Jan.–Mar. 1993.

Grisby, Jill S., "Paths for Future Population Aging." *Gerontologist* 31(2): 195–203, Apr. 1991.

Hamarat, E.; Thompson, D.; Aysan, F.; Steele, D.; Matheny, K.; and Simons, C. "Age Differences in Coping Resources and Satisfaction with Life among Middle-Aged, Young-Old, and Oldest-Old

Adults." *The Journal of Genetic Psychology; Child Behavior, Animal Behavior, And Comparative Psychology* 163(3): 360–7, Sept. 2002.

Hooyman, Nancy R., and Kiyak, H. Asuman. *Social Gerontology: A Multidisciplinary Perspective*, 6th ed. Ramsey, NJ: Allyn and Bacon, 2001.

Kart, Cary S., and Kinney, Jennifer M. *The Realities of Aging: An Introduction to Gerontology* 6th ed. Ramsey, NJ: Allyn and Bacon, 2000.

Kertzer, David I., and Laslett, Peter, eds. *Aging in the Past: Demography, Society, and Old Age*. Studies in Demography, vol. 7. Berkeley: University of California Press, 1995.

Lagrand, L., and Rando, T. *Changing Patterns of Human Existence: Assumptions, Beliefs, and Coping with the Stress of Change*. Springfield, IL: Charles C. Thomas Publisher, 1988.

Longino, Charles F., Jr. "Myths of an Aging America." *American Demographics* 16(8): 36–42, Aug. 1994.

Markson, Elizabeth W. *Social Gerontology Today: An Introduction*. Los Angeles, CA: Roxbury Publishing Company, 2002.

Mogey, John, et al. "The Aged in the United States: Kinship and Household." From *Aiding and Aging: The Coming Crisis in Support for the Elderly by Kin and State*, Mogey, J., ed. Contribution to the Study of Aging, no. 17. New York: Greenwood Press, 1990, 49–79.

Reberger, Caroline; Hall, Sonja E.; and Criddle, Arthur R. "Is Hostel Care Good for You? Quality of Life Measures in Older People Moving into Residential Care." *Australasian Journal on Aging* 18(3): 145–9, Aug. 1999.

Rothenberg, Richard; Lentzner, Harold R.; and Parker, Robert A. "Population Aging Patterns: The Expansion of Mortality." *Journal of Gerontology: Social Sciences* 46(2): S66–S70, Mar. 1991.

Schumacher, J.; Gunzelmann, T.; and Brähler, E. "Life Satisfaction in Old Age: Differential Aspects and Influencing Factors." *Zeitschrift für Gerontopsychologie und -psychiatrie* 1, Heft 1, S. 1–17 Verlag Hans Huber, Bern, Switzerland, 1996.

U.S. Census Bureau. "The 65-Year and Over Population: 2000." www.census.gov/prod/2001pubs/c2kbr01-10.pdf.

U.S. Census Bureau. "Population Pyramid Data for 249 Countries." www.census.gov/ipc/www/idbpyr.html. April 2005.

U.S. Census Bureau. "Statistical Abstract of the United States." www.census.gov/prod/3/98pubs/98statab/sasec1.pdf. September 1998.

Resources

✿ ✿ ✿

Authors' Website

For more information about the topics covered in this book, visit the authors' website: www.lwnh.com.

For General Information and Statistics on Aging

AARP
(888) 687-2277
www.aarp.org
AARP describes itself as "a nonprofit membership organization of persons fifty and older dedicated to addressing members' needs and interests." The website offers a long-term-care insurance policy and other information on long-term care, including nursing homes and living centers.

National Center for Health Statistics
www.cdc.gov/nchs/default.htm
This page of the website for the Centers for Disease Control and Prevention provides statistics on aging and health.

To Locate and Research Nursing Homes

www.MyZiva.net
This website states as its purpose "to help you find and compare nursing homes." You can use it to locate a nursing home in your (or your parent's) area and also to see how individual nursing homes measured up during recent inspections, using government-issued guidelines.

The same website also offers a clear and simple discussion of how to pay for a nursing home. Go to the following page: www.myziva.net/essentials/howtopay.php.

For Long-Term-Care Information and Advocacy

www.longtermcarelink.net
This website features links to many other websites addressing all aspects of long-term care, including finances and help for caregivers. It also includes links to many state agencies for senior services (see below).

www.medicare.gov/LongTermCare/Static/Home.asp
This U.S. government website has information about how to work with Medicare when there are long-term-care needs.

ElderCare Rights Alliance
2626 E. 82nd St., Suite 230
Bloomington MN 55425
(952) 854-7304
(952) 854-8535, fax
www.eldercarerights.org
Although this organization focuses part of its efforts on being a clearinghouse for information about long-term care in Minnesota, it also provides quite a bit of information on long-term-care topics in general, including the important role of residents' councils and family councils in nursing homes.

National Council on the Aging
409 3rd St. SW, Suite 200
Washington DC 20024
(202) 479-1200
www.ncoa.org

WISE Senior Services
1527 4th St., Suite 250
Santa Monica CA 90401
(310) 394-9871
www.wiseseniorservices.org
This website addresses a wide range of senior-service needs. The organization also provides general senior advocacy for residents of Los Angeles County.

To Contact State Agencies

Many states operate websites for senior services and long-term-care oversight. Here is the URL for Montana's, for example:

www.dphhs.state.mt.us/sltc (Senior and Long-Term-Care Division of the Montana Department of Public Health and Human Services)

You can access these state agencies through the following website, which includes links to many states' websites for senior services and long-term-care ombudsmen:

www.longtermcarelink.net

To Report a Case of Elder Abuse

National Center on Elder Abuse
www.elderabusecenter.org/default.cfm
Contains links to websites providing contact information for all fifty states' elder-abuse hotlines.

For Caregivers

www.caregivers.com
Contains listings for caregivers' support groups, organized by state.

National Association for Home Care
228 7th St. NE
Washington DC 20003
(202) 547-7424
www.nahc.org

ElderCare Online
www.ec-online.net
Offers support and information for caregivers.

Online Support for All Issues Faced by Adult Children of Elderly Parents

groups.yahoo.com *or* groups.google.com
Search under such topics as "caregivers" or "eldercare" or "Alzheimer's" or "Parkinson's," etc., to find specific online support groups you may be interested in joining.

To Learn Skills for Interpersonal Communication and Emotional Literacy

Insight Seminars
(310) 315-9733 *or* (800) 311-8001
www.insightseminars.org
Provides training for enhancing personal and professional effectiveness. Seminars are offered in several states as well as internationally.

The University of Santa Monica
(310) 829-7402
www.gousm.edu
A private graduate school offering programs in spiritual psychology for life mastery. Classes are held one weekend per month and are attended by students from all over the world.

Index

❧ ❧ ❧

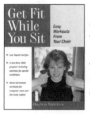
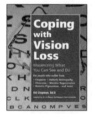
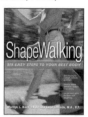
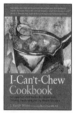
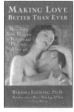